Subtle Energy Yoga
Volume 1: Foundations

Bench Yoga

For Easier Yoga and Enhanced Meditation

by Eric Armstrong

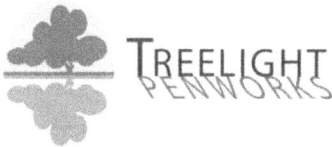

TREELIGHT
PENWORKS

SUBTLE ENERGY YOGA™

VOLUME 1
FOUNDATIONS

Bench Yoga

For Easier Yoga and Enhanced Meditation

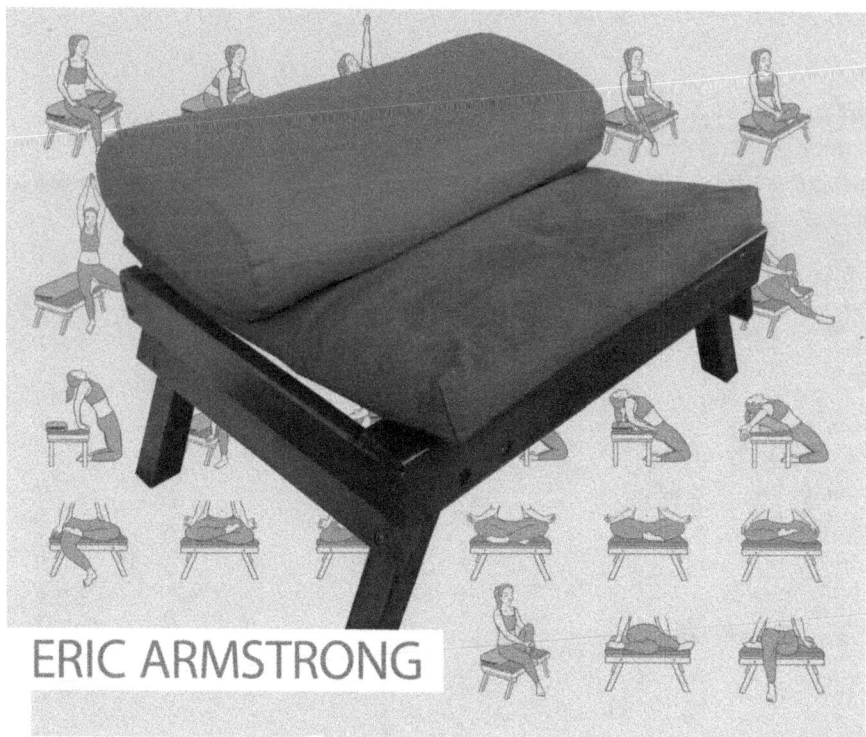

ERIC ARMSTRONG

Cover designed by George Foster.
Illustrations by Kathleen Karras and Leah Garza.
Copy editing by Alice Patrick.

ISBN 978-0-9972400-4-7 (print edition)

Published by TreeLight PenWorks
Mountain View, CA 94041
TreeLight.com

Printed and bound in the United States of America

Contents

Acknowledgements

A series of books that covers this much ground has its beginnings in the many wonderful lessons taught by so many great teachers:

- Great Grandmaster Dr. Tae Yun Kim, whose "tough love" martial arts program opened my heart in ways I never dreamed. She put up a mirror that forced me to see and acknowledge my real strengths—and my real weaknesses.

- Sifu Tony Wong and visiting master Chen Youze, who taught me the energy-flow principles and at least some of the applications of Chen-style Taiji (which originated as the Chen family's martial arts practice—as did all forms of Chinese Kung Fu in the day and age when it evolved.)

- My Ipsalu Tantra/Kriya Yoga teachers: Jan Robinson, Pat Henderson, Buddhyananda, Nayano Burdine, and Ipsalu founder, Bodhi Avinasha, whose energy-activation techniques gave me my first real experience of internal energy flows, and whose gentle nurturing opened my heart further.

- Shakti Padmini, who showed me how Yoga asanas can become a "tantric dance".

- Swami Yogananda for bringing "internal energy" Yoga to the West.

- His disciple Kriyananda, for writing an incredibly insightful book on Raja Yoga and for creating an intensive course that tears away the veils from the eyes. It was the "cherry on top" of my spiritual-growth sundae that allowed energy to flow freely, creating a newly-positive personality from cloth that had become charged with excessive negativity!

- The teachers in the lineage shared by the Ananda and Ipsalu traditions: Sri Yukteswar, Lahiri Masaya, and Babaji.

- Sunyata Saraswati, who combined Shivananda Tantra Kriya Yoga with Cobra Breath to create the powerful internal-energy practices that became the foundation of Ipsalu Tantra/Kriya Yoga.

o   Swami Asanganad Saraswati, a descendent of the Shivananda Yoga tradition, who gave the best Pranayama instruction I ever encountered, and who has assisted in my spiritual development in many other ways.

o   BKS Iyengar, who pioneered the use of supports in Yoga, inventing many for the purpose and making the practice of Yoga accessible for a population that grew up in the West.

o   Ennio Nimis from Italy, for the free online PDFs that share what he has learned about Kriya Yoga.

Beyond my "official" teachers, there are many others to thank as well.

My heartfelt gratitude to the faculty and staff of the Ananda center in Palo Alto CA: Vivekadevi, Kshama, Lakshmi, Navashen, Rammurti, Rose, Sita, Tandava. Their generosity of spirit is a continuing inspiration, and their willingness to respond to questions and the thoughts they shared during the Raja Yoga program sparked innumerable insights contained in the pages of this series.

But most of all, I owe a debt of gratitude to *Shanti*, who gave me the opportunity to undertake the Ananda Raja Yoga curriculum. She is the quintessential "Generous Spirit" who opened a huge door in my life.

My thanks to Helen Shaw, gentle-manipulation chiropractor and friend—a great listener and perfect sounding board, for helping divine answers to many a nagging question.

I also owe a debt of gratitude to the students of the Raja Yoga, Tantra, and Yoga courses I have attended. Their questions and observations sparked many additional insights—often rising in meditation in the weeks and years that followed, and subsequently recorded here.

Thanks as well to Alex Derevin and Julie Hsieh, my "Zombies Anonymous" buddies who helped to make introductory videos.

Finally, I am of course *deeply* indebted to my reviewers, and to the people whose efforts helped bring this book to fruition: My ever-patient illustrators: Leah Garza who created the first set of drawings for the Quick Start guide (reused here), and Kathleen Karras who did the bulk of the drawings, as well as cover designer George Foster and copy editor Alice Patrick. Their valuable contributions during the preparation of this book added greatly to its quality.

Preface

I have long been a fan of Yoga, just about forever. My love affair began in High School, when I read The Yoga System of Health and Relief from Tension, by Yogi Vithaldis. It was a slim volume, but it was chock full of details—not just on Yoga poses, or *asanas*, but many of the more esoteric practices, including *pranayama* (breathing) and internal cleansing rituals.

That book opened my eyes to a whole new way of looking at the world. It is my hope that this one will do something similar for you.

You see, while being a fan of the Yoga *concept*, I've been a lot less enchanted with the "gymnastics" Yoga taught in the West. Don't get me wrong. As a former athlete and coach, I have great admiration for physical fitness and dexterity. I would certainly do those gymnastics classes myself, if I could! But the fact of the matter is that if I try to do an entire hour of such things, I'm wiped out for a least a day afterward.

So when I go to a normal Yoga class, I wind up spending a lot of time sitting in meditation between poses! (Paradoxically, the kind of "Yoga Bootcamp" class where people go from "High Plank" to "Low Plank" a dozen times (i.e. push ups!) works well for me. I hate to miss an asana. But I can happily sit out the push ups. So I just sit, meditating away.)

At bottom, I am a fan of a gentler, more *meditative* kind of Yoga. I've noticed that a Yoga pose done right is done right at your personal *edge*— where you stretch enough to feel it, but not so much it hurts. (You'll find out more about that in the section on The Secret of Yoga.)

When you're working at that boundary, there is a small release of energy when you come out of the pose. It's small—barely a trickle. But once you become of aware of energy flows, it's something you can *feel*.

That awareness turns out to be the antidote for the competitive streak that forces me to practice in a class with my eyes closed! (If the person next to me is doing "better", I try too hard. If they're "not doing as well", I get all arrogant and superior. Neither mental state is of any use for that energy release.)

Of course, pranayama generates even stronger internal energy flows, and the kind of internal chakra-opening exercises I cover in subsequent books release flows that are stronger still. Nevertheless, the internal energy flow that comes from a pose done *right*—that is, right at your edge—are palpable.

In short, if you are working at your personal boundary, you are getting an internal-energy benefit from the practice. That is *Yoga done right*, in my book. Because that little flow, whether you are aware of it or not, is the *key* to a positive and joyful state of being. It's what makes the practice so worthwhile!

If you're a beginner, you get that flow from a very small movement. If you've been doing it a while, you need to stretch much further to get it.

It's exactly the same with a runner or weight lifter. To get the same "high" from the practice, you wind up doing more. And that's a good thing! But the point is that whether you go deep or shallow is only an indication of *how long* you have been practicing that particular pose.

That is an important concept to understand. The depth of your pose is *not* a measure of how much benefit you have derived from it. Because internally, stretching an inch may be giving you the exact same benefit as someone who is stretching a mile!

So one of my goals is to introduce a gentler, kinder, more meditative kind of Yoga. Another is to introduce the *Yoga Meditation Bench*—a sitting bench that makes it easier to practice Yoga (a boon for many of us), and that makes it possible to sit better and meditate more comfortably.

Because, while Child Pose is great in many ways, I want to encourage people to *sit in meditation*—before, during, and after their asana practice!

The bench gives you a way to sit comfortably today, regardless of your flexibility. At the same time, it gives you a way to *make progress toward more advanced positions*, up to and including Lotus Pose. So a Bench Yoga practice can not only make a Yoga practice easier and more accessible, it can also help to lengthen and deepen your meditations.

Once you begin to experience internal energy flows, those meditations become increasingly positive, uplifting experiences. In a word, they become *joyful*. You wind up practicing every day, because you *want* to.

Meditation shouldn't be something you have to *make* yourself do. I mean, it takes a lot of willpower to make yourself sit still for 20 minutes, bored out of your skull, trying not to think of anything! Instead, meditation should be something you *can't wait* to do—because you enjoy it.

That is the kind of practice I want to share in this series of books. Because *that* is when we make progress, as a species. That is how we grow towards something better—*together*.

This book lays the foundation, by using a sitting bench to create a form of Yoga that anyone can do—a form of Yoga that leads to better sitting positions, the experience of internal energy flows, and deeper meditations.

—Eric Armstrong, Mountain View, CA

About the Subtle Energy Yoga Series

Here are the current and planned volumes in the series:

Volume 1: Foundations

Bench Yoga

A Starter's Guide to Easier Yoga and Enhanced Meditation.

Bench Yoga is a quiet, meditative kind of yoga, with frequent meditation breaks. It emphasizes the specific kinds of strength and flexibility required to sit for meditation, and includes internal "energy flow" practices that bring a smile to your face and joy to your heart. This volume introduces the sitting bench, shows how to use it in your practice, and introduces you to preliminary "subtle energy" practices.

Volume 2: Awakening

The Yoga of Meditation

Sit long, Sit Strong, Meditate Better.

A deeper investigation of Yoga, sitting posture, and meditation. The principles of posture are explained, coupled with strengthening and stretching exercises that make it possible to achieve and maintain it. Readers of Bench Yoga will find much that is familiar, but also much that is new. This volume is ideal for traditional yoga practitioners. The practices it describes can be employed as part of a "normal" yoga practice.

Volume 3: Expanding

The Yoga of Internal Energy

Experience the joy of internal energy flows!

From chakra expansion to bandha contraction, from stretching a muscle to squeezing it, traditional spiritual practices have developed a variety of techniques to increase internal energy, and to get it flowing. This volume explores the subtle internal practices from those traditions—practices that are all but invisible to the naked eye, but which are incredibly effective tools for positive attitudes and energetic living!

Volume 4: Living in Joy

The New Science of Energy / The Energy Yoga Lifestyle

Ultimately, all of the energy that is available to us comes from the sun. (Even the wind and waves result from the influence of the sun!) An internal energy flow is a cascade of electrons that can be felt, the same way you can see light emanating from a lightbulb and feel heat from the wire leading to it. The lifestyle practices from all traditional spiritual practices can be understood as ones that maximize internal energy. This volume explores the latest findings in science of bioelectricity and shows how to apply them to daily life—starting with the breath and diet, and continuing with many other practices.

Introduction

The "sitting bench" actually has an ancient tradition behind it. In this section, we'll talk about its history and its many uses.

History of the Sitting Bench

As mentioned in the preface, I discovered the value of such a bench while sitting on the edge of my futon to meditate. Knee injuries hampered my ability to sit on the floor, but I didn't want to be confined to a chair for the rest of my life. The futon gave me a comfortable way to sit that also allowed me to *progress*.

But the futon I was using, with its serendipitously pulled-back cushion, was only really ideal for one leg! After a year, that leg had become quite flexible. But my weaker leg was lagging behind. So I began to look for a bench with the dimensions I needed. Not finding one, I resolved to build it!

Along the way, I did an image-search, starting with images of Shiva sitting on a bench. The search revealed *many* saints and gods from India sitting on a bench (or *throne*), with one leg up, and one leg down. It's a natural position!

This one is a huge sculpture in Kailasagiri, a hilltop park in Visakhapatnam, India:

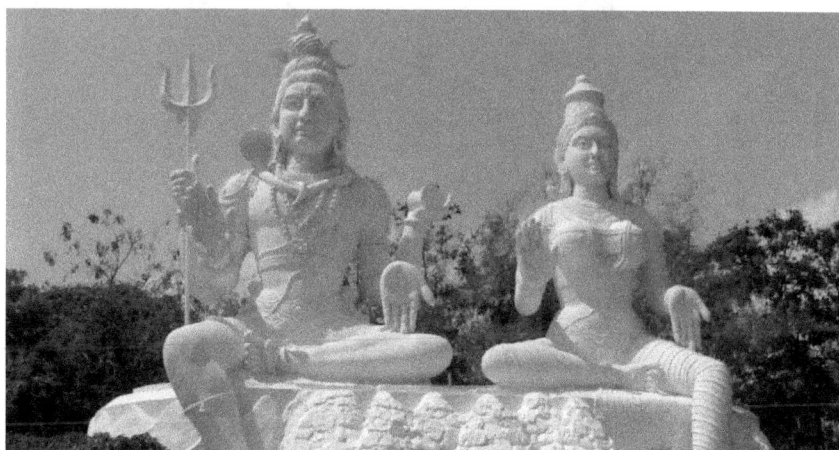

This sculpture is in the Metropolitan Museum of Art in New York:

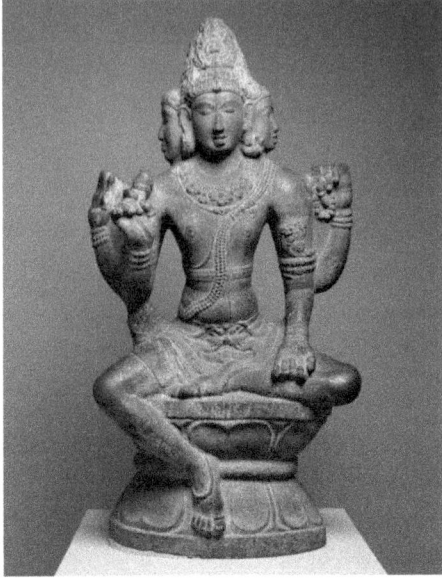

As is this one:

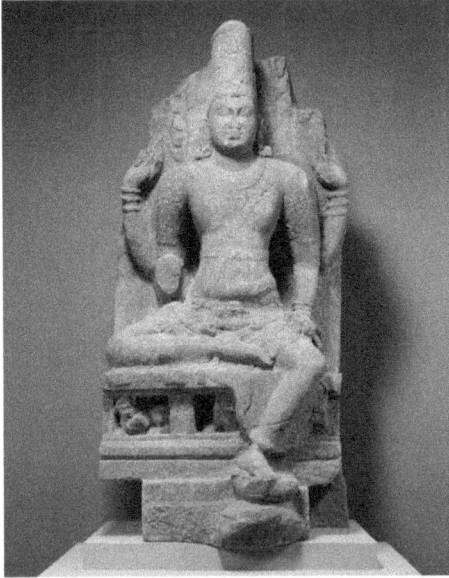

Here's one of Lakshmi:

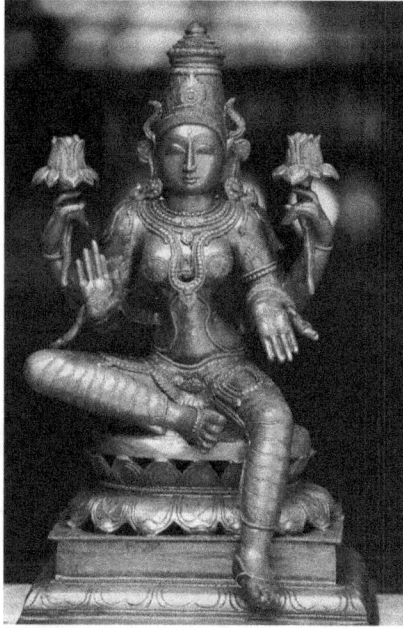

This one is in the British museum...

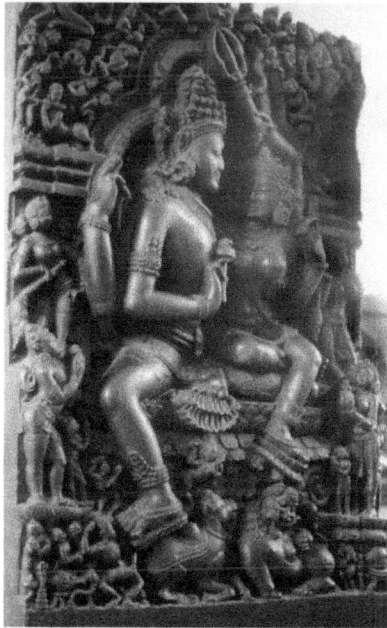

This picture shows Sri Dakshinamurthy, from the National Museum of India, where "*dakshina* means buddhi (knowledge) through which Shiva (who is Brahman) can be known".

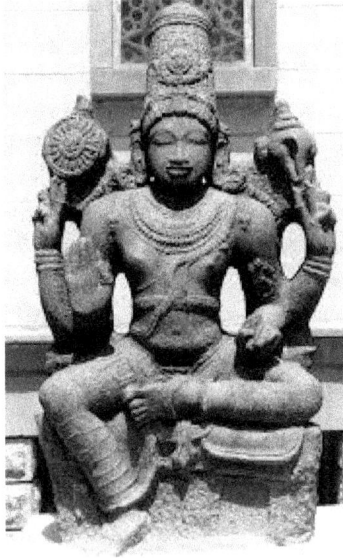

This drawing shows Shiva sitting on a kneeling cow...

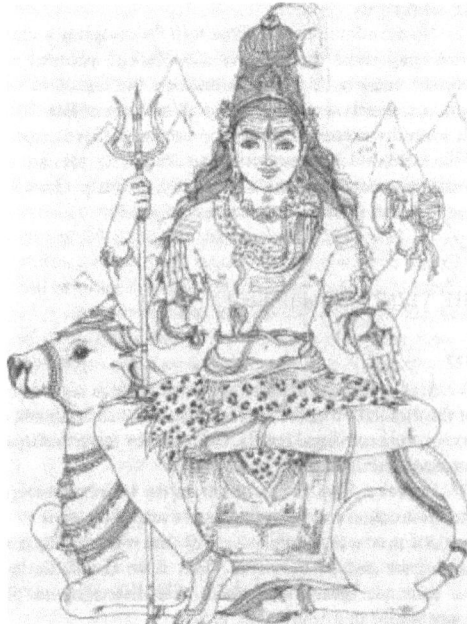

Here, Shiva is on a tree stump, foot on the head of the tiger skin:

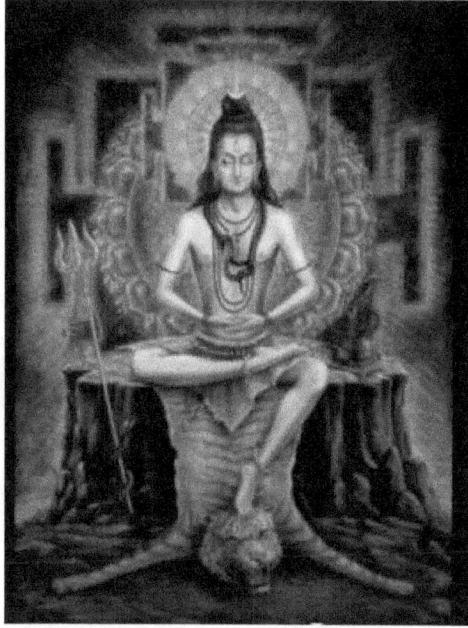

Here, guru Vasishta is in discussion with Brahma:

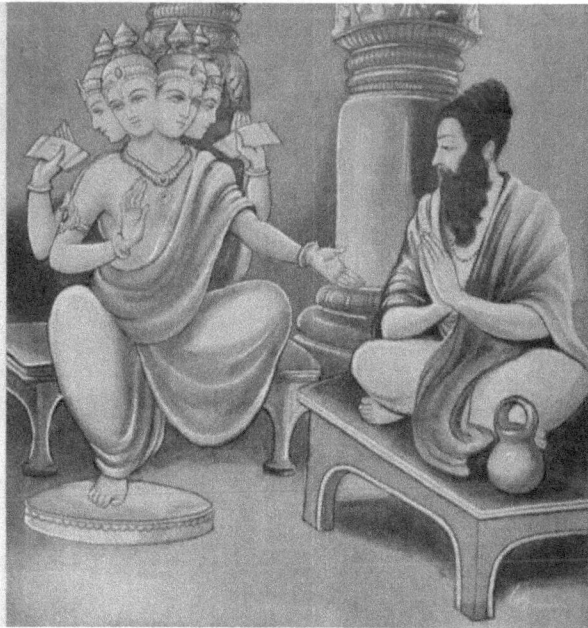

And just for a change of pace, here's one of Narasimha, Vishnu's man/lion avatar, sitting with one foot down and one knee raised:

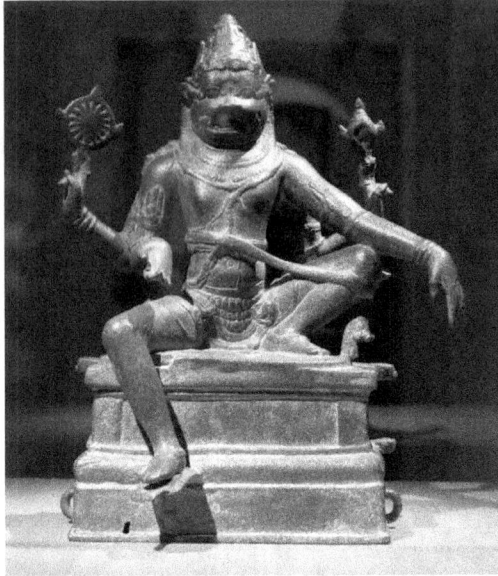

With so *many* ancient depictions of people sitting in that matter, it seems clear that it used to be a common practice. But virtually no one sits that way these days. I am forced to conclude that people *used* to sit in that manner, but then got so comfortable sitting on the floor that the tradition was eventually forgotten!

At any rate, perhaps one or more of those images were lingering in my mind the day I was sitting on the edge of my futon, and was inspired to sit in that manner. Perhaps my inspiration to create a meditation bench modeled on that idea came from Shiva (my personal deity). Wherever the inspiration came from, I was inspired to create a bench that made it possible to sit in that manner.

The next step was to come up with a name for it. "Shiva Seat" came to mind, mostly because Shiva is the deity I resonate with most, and because "Shiva" and "Seat" go together so well. Then, when I searched for images, I found Shiva to be sitting in that very manner, quite often!

Note:
Interestingly, "In Yogic tradition, Shiva is not a God. He is

called the Aadhi Yogi, Asdhi Bagawan (in Tamil), Aadi Devudu (in Telugu), Batara Guru (in Indonesia and Java). He is the first guru, and created the first spiritual path several millennium before any organized religion was formed."
http://www.ajithkumar.cc/sivam/shiva-buddha-and-eastern-atheism/

So, in case you were worried, you're not pretending to be a God, or taking on airs by sitting on a throne. You're just sitting the way the original teachers used to sit!

The trouble was, "sitting shiva" in the Jewish tradition means holding a wake. So, much as I loved the name, I was forced to discard it. (There's a lot of meditation in the Jewish tradition, too!) I finally settled on "TreeLight Yoga Bench", as a short version of the longer "Yoga/Meditation Bench" I discuss on my website, TreeLight.com.

As for which leg to have on the bench when sitting with one leg down, here is a link to a **Quora story** that says having the left leg up promotes masculine energies, while the right leg promotes feminine. I'm not sure I buy any of it, but it is interesting. (And luckily for me, my left leg is more flexible, so I typically sit with my left leg up!)
https://www.quora.com/How-does-lord-Shiva-sit-with-one-leg-on-the-stone-and-other-hanging-Is-there-a-yogic-or-a-spiritual-significance-to-it

The Many Uses of the Sitting Bench

The Yoga/Meditation Bench has many uses: For sitting and meditating, to improve your sitting capacity, for Yoga, and for rehabilitation. It just may be the best investment you ever make!

For Sitting and Meditating

Using the TreeLight Yoga/Meditation bench (or one of similar dimensions):

○   You can sit with the perfect upright posture that eliminates back pain.

○   Sitting in that manner for short periods each day helps you develop the strength you need to *maintain* that posture.

○   You can choose one of *many* sitting positions.

○   It's easy to get up and down. (You can even use Yoga Blocks for arm rests!)

○   You can start as easily as sitting in a chair, and gradually progress to more advanced positions.

○   You can change positions whenever you need to.

Sit straight. Meditate. Grow into Lotus.

To Grow into Lotus

If you can sit in a chair, you can sit on the TreeLight Yoga bench—*today*. And you can use a variety of specialized asanas and strengthening techniques to *bring Lotus Pose within your grasp*.

I myself was a card-carrying member of the terminally-inflexible club! And I can tell from personal experience that the regular use of the bench can take you:

From Human Brick to Human Pretzel

It can get you closer, at least. And it can get you there more quickly than any other way.

To Eliminate Back Pain

Back-support cushions create good posture, which alleviates many pains. But, at the very same time, *they weaken the muscles you need* to maintain that posture. So over time, you get more and more uncomfortable *everywhere else* in your life, whether standing, sitting, or walking.

If you are sitting for long hours, or you are experiencing great pain, then by all means use the back-support devices whenever you need them.

But at the same time, make it habit to *sit on the bench* each day. Build up to 20 minutes at a time, changing positions as often as you need to in order to keep your legs comfortable.

Sit Long, Sit Strong

You can do it while meditating, reading, sewing, knitting, playing music, or watching TV. Or do it at the computer. From the standpoint of building "sitting strength", it doesn't really matter *what* you're doing—just sitting on the bench for extended periods of time will do several important things:

1. In time, your neuromuscular system will identify *the point of maximum balance*, where it takes *minimal effort* to remain upright.

2. Once it does, your neuromuscular system will *automatically assume that position*, whenever and wherever it can.

3. You will *gradually develop strength and flexibility* in the areas that need it—a combination of capabilities that, in addition to having you sitting straighter and more comfortably, will have you standing taller and even sleeping better.

That practice all by itself will build the strength to maintain *back comfort all day long*. But you can go even further to build your sitting strength, and to become a "strong sitter", by doing *exercises* designed to strengthen the muscles you need and *asanas* (stretching exercises) that increase the specialized flexibility required for sitting, so your muscles don't have to work as hard!

We'll talk about those exercises and asanas in coming chapters.

To Improve Your "Sitting Strength"

Over time, your sitting strength and flexibility will improve, simply by virtue of the fact that you have been able to spend time in a position that is somewhat more advanced than sitting in a chair.

The Longer You Sit, the Stronger you Get

For a faster rate of progress, use the bench for the Sitting-Position Asanas that are so important for flexibility in the hip, groin, and legs.

You can also do the Sit Strengtheners—a series of exercises that build the strength you need in the back, neck, and core. Those exercises are devoted to sitting strength. Using them will improve your posture rapidly, and they will generate the kind of internal energy flows that make meditation a positively joyful experience.

Of course, several of the standard Yoga asanas help to build sitting strength as well. The trick is to know which ones! See the Build Great Posture section for a plan that selects the practices that contribute directly to your sitting strength.

For Yoga and Rehabilitation

The specialized asanas and exercises enabled by the bench can be used for recovery and rehabilitation after injury or surgery. In addition, the bench can be used for a variety of Yoga asanas—bringing the health-giving benefits to many who would otherwise be unable to participate in a Yoga program.

Yoga for Everyone. Isolate the Areas that Need Work.

To achieve those goals:

1. Most importantly, do the sitting position asanas to develop the *flexibility* needed in the hips, groin, and legs. In time, those asanas will move you toward Lotus Pose.

2. Although it is not exactly "Yoga" as we commonly think of it, consider doing the strengthening exercises, as well (the "Sit Strengtheners"). Those exercises build strength where it is needed in the neck, back, and core to help you to maintain an upright posture.

3. There are also a variety of ways in which the bench can help you perform many of the Standard Asanas.

Important Principles

Before going any further, let's take a moment to answer a couple of important questions:

- What is an *asana*?
- What is the *secret* of yoga?
- What is *Bench Yoga*?

What is an "Asana"?

Let's start by clarifying what we mean by the word "asana".

- Both in India and in the West, an *asana* is a Yoga pose or position.
- In Hindi, the word *asan(a)* also means "place where you sit".
- So it's fair to assume that the original meaning of *asana* was "things you do while sitting, for the purpose of sitting *better*". In other words: *Practices intended to enhance meditation* (!).
- Further, the ancient scholar Patanjali (*pah-**tahn**-jah-lee*) defines an asana as "a position you can reside in, comfortably, for a lengthy period of time". In other wors, it's a position you can be in *joyfully*, with a smile on your face!
- In its essence, then, an *asana* is any position you can use for meditation!

All of which brings us to an important principle:

If you're doing Yoga with a Smile,
You're doing it Right.

Note:
The Shivananda Yoga tradition leans heavily on Patanjali and other ancient Vedic texts—pretty much to the exclusion of everything else, so it's as "pure" as a tradition can get. I have added a lot to that practice, but the ability to reference the original, unalloyed sources is a precious gift. I was fortunate enough to be introduced to that source of wisdom by a

visiting teacher, Swami Asanganand Saraswati, who tours the U.S. once a year introducing the finer points of Yoga. (For more information, see the Resources.)

The Secret of Yoga

The secret of Yoga is that the whole point of the exercise boils down to one thing: *energy flows*.

The strongest energy flows are stimulated by very small muscular contractions along the spine—the *bandhas* and *mudras* of Yoga. You'll be learning a lot more about them in later parts of the Subtle Energy Yoga series.

Strong energy flows are also stimulated by *pranayama* ("energy breathing" exercises). All of those energy-releasing activities are a great prelude to meditation. The energy they release is positive, fulfilling, and uplifting. In a word, they bring you closer to the awesome power and wisdom of the universe—or God, if that is the word you choose to use.

The Secret of Yoga is Energy Flows.

But perhaps an unsung benefit of Yoga *asana* is that those postures also generate energy flows!

Note:
There are ways to make asanas even more effective, with subtle movements—at times all but invisible to the naked eye—that produce even stronger energy flows. Those, too, are introduced in this book, with more information coming in future installments in this series.

Energy Flows

The energy released by asana is small compared to that released by energy-focused activities like mudras, bandhas, and pranayama. But it is real. So in a sense, even large physical movements produce a *subtle* kind of energy flow.

The smaller, more tightly-focused muscular contractions along the spine release larger amounts of energy—but you may not even notice it, unless you're looking for it. (All you know is that you feel good, which is why so many people are so attracted to Yoga!)

But once you become aware of energy sensations then, when you release an asana, you notice a tiny energy surge.

Physical asanas release energy, too!

That surge occurs when you do stretch and strengthen "just the right amount".

The next question of course, is: How much is "just right"?

The answer is highly personal, but it always lies between too little (not enough) and too much. If you don't stretch far enough, you don't get any effect. If you stretch too far and it becomes painful, the energy surge is dwarfed by the pain.

The same is true for the many *strengthening* moves in a Yoga asana practice. If you don't do enough, you don't get much in the way of benefit. If you do too much, you get sore. (You know you've done too much if it takes most of the next day to recover!)

Reveling in Your Limitations

That energy surge occurs right at your *personal limit*: The area between too little and too much. If you are working at that limit, you are getting the benefit. (How do you know? You feel it, but you're still smiling!)

"Just enough" is when you feel it,
but you are still smiling.

But here's the real key: *Everyone is getting the same surge.*

If you're a beginner, you get it by bending an inch. If you're an experienced practitioner, you get it by bending a yard.

The fact is this: *Your body adapts.* So if you got that energy flow by bending an inch today, next week you'll need to bend an inch and a half.

It's just like weight lifting, or running. Each of those activities produces a nice release of pleasurable endorphins. If you're lifting weights, in time you need to lift more to get the same release. When running, you find that you need to run longer, or faster.

You *can* lift more or run longer, because your body adapted. But you *want* to, because you enjoyed the energy release. That's why exercise is called a "positive addiction". It's addictive, certainly. But it's also good for you. So it's *positive*.

But the real point of this section is this: It doesn't matter how far you go—what matters is the *energy* you feel. And *every* practitioner who is working at their limit feels the same amount of energy!

> *Every practitioner experiences the same*
> *energy flow, regardless of their level.*

That energy flow is what makes the practice enjoyable. When you feel it, it means you are obtaining maximum benefit, as well.

The Antidote for Competition

Perhaps you've heard that in a Yoga class you shouldn't be comparing yourself to others. But it's hard not to, right? I mean, especially if you have any kind of competitive streak. You just want to be doing as well as the person next to you!

But once you realize that the point of the exercise is an *energy flow*, competition becomes pointless. Because the fact is that you are getting the same energy flow at your limit that the beginner next to you is getting at an inch, and the advanced practitioner on the other side is getting at a yard.

In other words, the degree to which you can stretch is simply a measure of *how long* you have been doing the practice. If you've been doing it a long time, your limit is far. If not, it's short. But the fact of the matter is that everyone receives the same benefit.

> *Everyone gets the SAME benefit*
> *by working at their personal limit.*

What Is "Bench Yoga"?

Many Yoga practitioners know that the root word of "Yoga" means "yoke", or "union". In other words, the goal of Yoga is *union with the greater power and wisdom of the universe*, as known to you by whatever name you choose to use.

In other words, the goal of Yoga goes far beyond contortionist-level flexibility and gymnastic-level strength. Those things are great. Don't get me wrong. But they are *extraneous* to the primary goal!

"Bench Yoga" is the practice of using a bench to achieve that goal, with the *primary focus on sitting position and meditation*, and with a secondary focus on general health, strength, and flexibility.

Health is obviously important, and worth pursuing. That subject covers nutrition, lifestyle, daily activities, and sleep patterns, all of which lie outside the scope of "Bench Yoga" (to be covered in Volume 4 of this series).

Strength and flexibility are important, too. And the Bench Yoga program will help you get to where you can engage in more strenuous versions of those pursuits that focus on generalized strength and flexibility.

But the *primary focus* of Bench Yoga is on the strength and flexibility you need for *sitting*, so you can meditate longer and more deeply. So when you take into account that *asan* means "place where you sit", Bench Yoga is in a very real way a return to the *roots* of Yoga.

Bench Yoga: Returning Yoga to its Roots

Making or Buying a Yoga Meditation Bench

A meditation bench can be a fine piece of furniture or a lightweight, stackable unit. Or you can build your own. Whichever way you go, it's a good investment in your health and sanity!

Purchasing a Commercial Bench

The easiest way to get started, of course, is to purchase a commercially available Yoga Meditation Bench. The wooden furniture-style tends to be preferred for use at home, while the stackable-plastic version tends to be preferred for use in Yoga Studios, since it is lighter and less expensive. (And stackable. Did I mention stackable?)

You can also purchase cushions that go with the bench and other accessories that help to make it as useful as possible. Or, if you already have nicely "broken in" cushions you like, you can purchase the bench by itself and use your own cushions.

You can make your own, too, if you like. We will talk about that next. To purchase one, and for accessories, go to yogaBench.TreeLight.com.

Making a Custom Bench

If you are handy with tools, it is fairly easy to make your own sitting bench.

One advantage of making a custom bench is that you can make it the perfect size for your body. Of course, as with a standard chair, "one size fits most"—so the commercially available versions work for most everyone (and they save a lot of time and trouble).

The disadvantage is that your homemade version may be heavier than it needs to be and less portable than it could be, but if cost is an issue or you need special dimensions, then building your own is the way to go!

When done, the bench will look like the one shown on the next page.

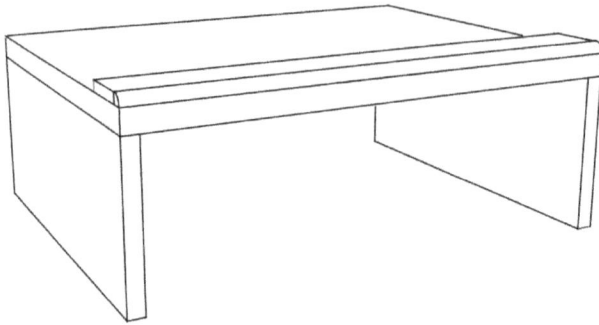

1. Start by building a "box" that is open at the front. (It can be open or closed at the rear).

2. Inexpensive plywood works great, or you can use other woods, if you prefer.

3. If you're 200 lbs or less, ½-inch plywood is fine. If you're over 300 lbs, ¾-inch plywood will work better. In the 200-300 lb range, ½-inch plywood may still be okay, but ¾-inch plywood is perfectly stiff (although it weighs more).

4. For the basic bench, all you really need are a top and two sides. They can be joined together with angle brackets, or using any joinery techniques you happen to be comfortable with.

5. The top will be 20 to 24 inches deep, front to back.

    - A taller user (6 feet and up) will find 24 inches more comfortable. A shorter user will find 20 inches to be deep enough.

    - It will ideally be 25 inches wide, so it sits *over* a Yoga Mat, rather than *on* it. (A Yoga Mat is 24 inches wide. At 25 inches wide, the bench sits over the mat without compressing it.)

6. The sides will have the same front-to-back dimension. The height will depend on the thickness of the top.

    - The top of the bench should be no more than 4 inches taller than a Yoga Block (which is 9 inches high, in its tallest orientation), and no less than an inch taller than the block.

    - So the top of the bench can be 10- to 13-inches tall.

- That way, the bench is at an intermediate height between a Yoga Block on the floor and one on the bench. And when you add seat cushions to it, the user is sitting at about the height of a normal chair (17 inches).

7. The real key is to add a *foot rail* at the open front of the bench. (Its importance will be explained later.)

    - The foot rail is a 2-1/2" strip of wood. A thickness of ½ inch is fine for a thin cushion (1 inch or less). For a thicker 2-inch cushion, a ¾ inch thickness is best.

    - It runs the length of the bench, right at the front edge.

    - If you have the tools, you can round-over the front edge, so your leg won't be resting on a sharp corner.

    - Or, for an alternative, set the strip of wood half an inch back from the front edge, then glue or tack a strip of half-inch, quarter round molding in the slot you created.

8. If you're following a video, it can help to add *a second foot rail*, at the back.

    - For a few asanas, you need to be facing the bench.

    - With a foot rail at the back of the bench, you can get behind it, move the seat cushion, and face the bench and the video (or teacher) at the same time, without having to turn your back to the instructor.

Adding Cushions for Sitting

To use the bench, you'll want to add cushions. I recommend these for sitting:

- Bean Products Zabuton, 24 x 24 x 2" – *base pad.*
- Bean Products Rectangular Bolster, 24 x 12 x 6" – *seat cushion.*

Those cushions, or ones of similar size that you favor, let you sit with the greatest comfort in positions that lead naturally and gracefully to Lotus Pose.

Getting Started

What you need to know about setting up and accessorizing.

Setting Up

The first thing to know is which way is front!

For Sitting and Meditating

Add cushions, and you're ready to sit.

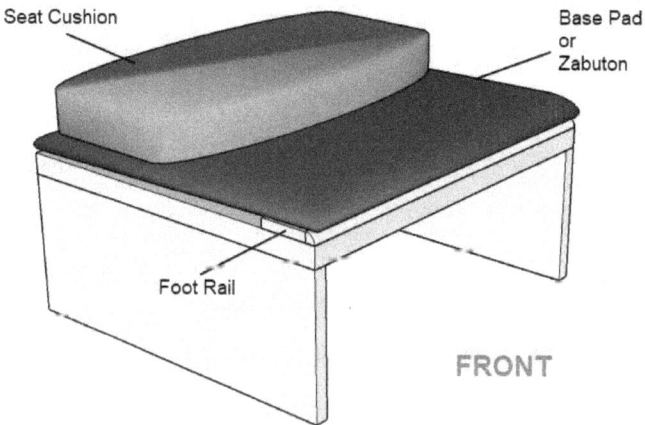

Seat Cushion

Base Pad
or
Zabuton

Foot Rail

FRONT

For Yoga

A single Yoga Block gives you seven levels of support for your Yoga poses, as shown in the figure on the following page.

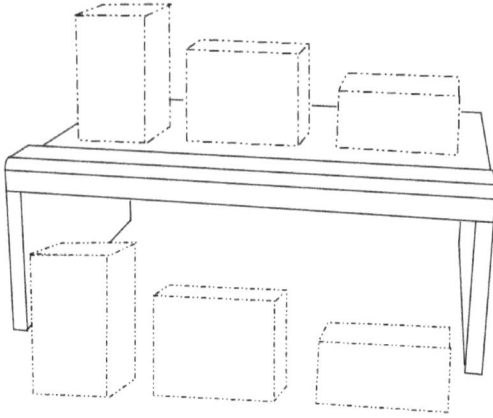

Notes:

- A bench that has a foot rail at front and at back is ideal when taking a class or following a video. You can then get behind the bench, make that the new front, and still see the instructor.
- Blocks can be placed on the base pad in front of the seat cushion. (There's no need to remove the cushions.)

Accessorizing

Helpful things to have on hand when you are using your bench.

Support Cushion

A half-size rectangular bolster finds many uses in Bench Yoga. It provides soft support for the back and chest in a variety of poses.

- Gayo Meditation Cushion, 15x10x5" (if available)
- YogaAccessories Cotton Meditation Pillow, 15x11x5"

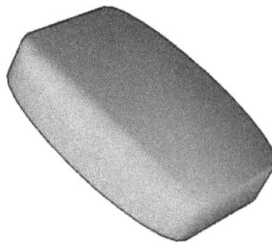

Four-Inch Yoga Blocks

You will also want a Yoga Block (two is ideal), for stretching poses. They come in handy, whether you are doing standard Yoga asanas or the special sitting asanas that improve your sitting flexibility.

One is sufficient, but two is ideal.

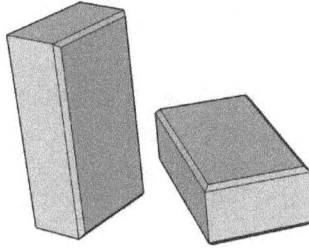

Cork Yoga Blocks are the best, in my view. They're lightweight, and very sturdy. You want 6 x 9 x 4" blocks, rather than the smaller 6 x 9 x 3" versions. You'll appreciate the extra stability when you have the block on its edge, and even more so when it is upright.

In combination with the bench, Yoga Blocks give you a range of support heights that go from the height of a normal chair down to the floor, so you always have support at the exact height that you need.

They can also be used to provide support for your thighs when sitting, and even sit on them, in some cases. They come in handy as arm rests, if you need a little help to get up and down from the bench. So they are pretty indispensable, in general.

Leg Cushion(s)

It also helps to have a small cushion or two to rest your thigh on, for when your knee is hovering several inches above the bench. It makes your position a lot more comfortable.

I've found that the wrist-pad cushions they sell for a computer mouse work quite well. You might need two of them, if they're small. I found a bean cushion that is the length of a small keyboard. It can be doubled over to make it taller, or left stretched out to keep it short.

Side Stand / Basket

A small stand next to the bench is great for a holding a pad and pen for notes, and the leg cushion, among other things. A small basket on the stand helps if you have multiple small items. For example, the basket on my stand holds:

○ **Mala Beads** – 108 beads on a string, used for my all-too infrequent *mantra* practice (chanting).

○ **Red Light headlamp** – I like to meditate in the middle of the night, when it's super quiet. If I need to jot down a note, or get a glass of water, the red light lets me do it without disturbing my night vision—so the world doesn't suddenly go *black* when I turn off the light.

○ **Glasses** – For when I want to see what I'm writing or refer to a book.

○ **Egg Timer** – A quiet one, for the infrequent occasions when I want to do something for a particular amount of time.

Using the Yoga Meditation Bench

The right cushions keeps you comfortable, but they also tilt your pelvis at just the angle to produce the ideal sitting position.

Orienting the Bench

The bench is open at the front and back, with legs on the sides. One end of the bench also has a *foot rail*—a small strip a couple of inches wide that rises half an inch above the bench surface. (For classes and video instruction, it helps to have a bench that has a foot rail at both the front and the back, so you don't have to turn the bench around.)

That foot rail identifies the *front* of the bench. It serves several important purposes:

1. Calf support.

   - The wide, flat surface on top supports the calf when the lower leg is on the bench.

   - Of course, the bench would do that as well, but in that case there would be more pressure on the foot—which brings us to the other two purposes for the foot rail.

2. Ankle-bone relief for a bent ankle.

   - When the ankle is bent, the calf and the edge of the foot are on the foot rail.

   - Because the foot and calf are supported, the heel has no weight on it, so it hovers over the bench, at about the same height as the foot rail. It may even be rotated slightly, so that the heel winds up angled *above* the height of the foot rail.

   - In either case, the ankle bone never touches the bench, so there is no pressure on it. At most, it creates a small depression in the cushion, which becomes a soft cradle for that bone.

3. Foot brace for a straight ankle.

- When the ankle is straight, the lower leg can be rotated slightly so the top of the foot and the top of the small toes are on the bench, behind the foot rail.

- In that position, the ankle bone is not pressing into the bench, the arch of the foot cradles the bottom of the other thigh, and the foot rail helps to keep the foot from sliding off the bench.

- Because the thigh extends outward from the seat cushion, it doesn't exert any pressure on the foot, so the position is comfortable to maintain.

- At the same time, it encourages the slight rotation of the lower leg that makes the position so comfortable—a rotation that is *needed* for Lotus Pose.

- The top of the foot also rests against the foot rail. But because of the cushion, there is no sensation of pressure.

Cushioning the Bench

For sitting comfortably for the seated asanas, and for many of the back-bend asanas, the right cushions make a big difference.

Base Cushion

The base cushion gives your lower leg a soft surface to rest on. It is fairly thin however (or very soft), so that the foot rail still works its magic.

Seat Cushion

A standard square Yoga bolster is 6 inches tall, so it works well as a seat cushion. That is a comfortable height for most, but smaller users may find that a shorter seat cushion makes it easier for their knees to reach the bench. Similarly, more flexible users may find that their knees comfortably reach the bench even with a short cushion.

If the seat cushion is placed 6 inches back from the front of the bench, there is plenty of room to bring one foot up on the bench. Placed 9 inches back, there is room for both feet.

The difference in height between the seat cushion and the base pad means that when you are sitting, your thighs extend from your hips at a comfortable 15-degree angle—about the same angle as when you are sitting on a gentle slope.

That angle encourages a slight forward tilt of the pelvis that centers your back over the tripod created by your legs. When your back is upright and your head balanced on top of your spine, you are centered in that position and very stable.

Because that angle is so desirable for the comfort of the back, many chairs have been designed with a sloping surface. But with the bench, you can vary the angle to suit your anatomy, and there is no tendency to slide forward (and slide off!) so you don't experience the strain on your thighs that occurs when you attempt to maintain your position on a sloping surface.

Support Cushion(s)

To sit comfortably, you need three points of support. One is the seat cushion you're sitting on. The other two are for the knees, ideally, or with support at a point midway up the calf or thigh of the leg, which achieves the same goal.

The three points of support create a *stable tripod*. When your legs are comfortable in that tripod, and your back is upright and balanced over it, you are "sitting strong", and it will be much easier to meditate.

When one foot is on the ground, the foot itself can be the third support. But even better, the thigh can be angled outward until the knee is resting on the bench, or until the thigh is resting on the ball of the other foot.

In fact, once you find that position, you'll notice that when the thigh rests on the ball of the foot, it extends from there over the arch of the foot, and runs *behind* the heel, so there is little pressure on the foot, and none on the heel. (That is the purpose of the foot-position progression covered in the next section.)

However, it is often the case that until sufficient flexibility is acquired, one knee just doesn't want to go down as far as the bench!

In that case, a small leg cushion can be useful. It can be placed under the thigh to give you the support you need for that leg. Or, when sitting with both legs up on the bench in poses we will talk about later, the cushion can be placed on the foot of the bottom leg, to provide a taller support for the leg above it.

Ideally, the support cushion will give you some flexibility in size. For example, I have a wrist-support cushion for typing at the keyboard that contains gel beads. There is enough space in that cushion that it can be doubled over, producing two support-heights for the price of one.

Changing Your Angle

When sitting with both legs up on the bench, a leg cushion is often necessary. But one of the advantages of the bench is that you can sit with *one* leg up. When you do, and the knee doesn't want to go all the way down to the bench, you can get extra support for the thigh merely by changing your angle:

1. You can change the angle of the seat cushion so it supports more of your thigh. For example, if your right foot is up, you can angle the cushion so the right end is closer to the front of the bench.

2. Rather than angling the cushion, you can simply angle your body so you are facing slightly to the right.

With either adjustment, part of the cushion is under your thigh, as well as your backside. So even if the knee isn't making it all the way down to the bench, it isn't under any pressure to do so. You're sitting comfortably.

You may also find that moving your knee closer to your centerline makes it more comfortable. Moving it farther out to the side, on the other hand, increases the pelvic tilt that makes your *back* comfortable—but it can result in noticeably more pressure on the knee, if it isn't resting comfortably on the bench.

Finding Comfort and Balance

The first thing to do is to sit on the bench and find your point of balance.

You can sit with both feet on the floor, as though you were in a chair— but many people have a tendency to slump when they do that. Alternatively, you can sit with both feet on the bench, as though you were sitting on the floor—something that works well only if you're already pretty flexible.

For most people, the ideal sitting position has one foot up on the bench and the other on the floor. There is just something about that position that encourages natural spine alignment. Perhaps that's why India has so many sculptures and pictures of ancient gods, gurus, and disciples sitting in exactly that manner.

Finding Foot Comfort

Sit with one foot up on the bench. The first thing to notice is that, because you are sitting on the seat cushion, your other thigh extends *over* the foot that is on the bench. That lets you straighten your ankle, so it doesn't have to be bent.

Next, notice how the *foot rail* at the front of the bench helps to make you more comfortable. If your ankle is straight, your foot can lean against it. And if your flexibility is limited, it helps to keep your foot from sliding away from you and off the bench.

But notice that it makes things more comfortable even if your ankle is bent—something you'll normally do when sitting in "Easy" Pose, for example. (It's easy to get into. It's just not all that easy to maintain.)

Try it now. Bend your ankle, and rest the edge of the foot on the rail at the front of the bench. Notice how the entire weight of the leg is supported by the calf and the edge of the foot, both of which are on that rail.

Now notice the ankle bone! It is hovering in air, just behind the rail. It puts a little depression in the base pad, but it is nowhere near the top of the bench. That is one of the secrets of the comfort you get when sitting on the bench!

Finding the Center of Your Tripod

The bench makes it possible to sit with one foot up, and it makes that foot as comfortable as can be. But perhaps the most important reason for sitting with one foot up is that helps you find your ideal point of balance—an upright posture that feels weightless, so it is easy to maintain, and which at the same time allows subtle internal energy flows to take place within your body. (You may or may not be aware of them, at the moment. If not, just trust me for now!)

Take a moment now to find that balance.

Start by identifying the center of your tripod:

1. Notice that your knees, thighs, and backside form a triangle.
2. Put the palm of one hand on your knee, and back of the other hand on your backside.
3. Be aware of the space between your hands.
4. Mentally identify the *halfway point* between them.
5. Put a finger at that point.

Notice that the halfway point is only a few inches in front of your torso. We're used to looking with our eyes. So what we *see* as halfway is much further forward than the *actual* halfway point. This exercise helps you identify the real center of your tripod.

Finding Your Posture

Next, practice centering yourself:

1. Lift upwards through the spine, as though someone was pulling your head straight up.
2. Lean forward, until your head is over the center point.
3. Without moving your lower back, raise your head and upper back so they are upright, rather than leaning forward.

Finding the Point of Balance

You have now achieved the ideal posture, but you are probably feeling a little strain in your back from the forward lean.

Continuing:

4. Keeping your back in that semi-arched position, lean back slightly until the sense of strain goes away.
5. At this point, the tip of your nose is at or just behind the center point.

It may take some practice, but eventually you will discover a sense of *weightlessness*. You get that feeling when the weight of your torso is perfectly balanced over your spine, and your muscles are doing very little work to stay upright.

That is your point of balance.

Getting There Quickly

Once you have identified your point of balance, your body will begin to remember it. Once you learn it, you can get there more quickly with this 2-step process:

1. Tilt your pelvis forward.
2. Stretch upward.

This subtle movement brings your head and torso over the center of the tripod and puts your back in a perfectly upright, *natural* position.

Note:

In that position, your back isn't exactly "neutral", due to the small curve in your lower back—but that "neutral" position is artificial. It also collapses your chest and shoulders, making it harder to breathe. Finally, that slight collapse brings your head forward, which makes the neck work harder to keep your head balanced over your spine.

Getting There Automatically

Sitting this way even for a short period of time helps to train your neuromuscular system. You may or may not know it, but your body is the smartest, most adaptive machine on the planet! When it finds a way to reduce strain and effort, it does so—*automatically.*

So even if you aren't consciously aware of it, your body is beginning to learn how to sit, *effortlessly.* The more you do it, the more it becomes your body's preferred position—a position it will adopt whenever and wherever it can.

And your body will automatically maintain that posture, for as long as your musculature is strong enough to maintain it. (It's *almost* effortless. It requires minimal muscular effort—but it requires that effort in muscles you may not be using regularly!)

With that posture comes a renewed sense of confidence and respect from others. All good things, of course. But the *real* reason for doing it is that it helps you sit better—at work, and in meditation.

Getting Better

At the outset, your ability to sit comfortably at the point of balance will be limited by your hip and groin flexibility (needed to get into position) and by the strength of a few muscles.

Even if those muscles aren't doing a *lot,* they are still doing *something.* And sitting in this manner for even a few moments, you may be discovering muscles you didn't even know you had!

Fear not. You have taken an important first step. If you have found the point of balance, your neuromuscular system has begun to learn where it is and how to find it. That's huge.

The more you sit this way, the stronger and more flexible you will get, in precisely those areas where you *need* strength and flexibility to sit well. So if you do nothing else you will improve organically, in time.

We will do better than that, however. In this book, you'll learn asanas that develop your flexibility, as well as exercises that build to your strength.

Before we get to those, though, let's talk about the *many possible ways* you can sit on the bench.

Four Types of Sitting Position (11 positions, 45 variations)

Wow. Eleven basic sitting positions, and 45 variations on the themes. That's a lot! They can be divided into 4 categories:

1. Both feet on the floor.

2. One foot on the bench.

3. One knee raised.

4. Both feet on the bench.

In this section, we will cover the 11 different ways you can sit on the bench, and the *45 variations* of those positions—*not counting* hand positions (covered later), and *not counting* intermediate positions (also covered later), and without concern for which leg is on top.

In other words, when I say there are "45" variations of the 11 basic positions, I'm being conservative! There are many variations I'm not counting. The important message is that there are *many* ways to get comfortable on the bench—and when one position stops being comfortable, it's easy to change to another one.

How The Variations Were Counted

Since we have two legs and two feet, there are always two variations for any position that isn't totally symmetrical—one for the left foot and leg, and one for the right.

About the only sitting position that is really "symmetrical" is when both feet are on the floor. So that position has the smallest number of variations (5). The other positions all have left- and- right versions, which means the total number of variations is *twice* the number of variations that are available for one leg!

If we wanted to, then, we could consider "left leg on top" as one position, and "right leg on top" as another position—even if one position is a mirror image of the other. If we did that, we could really inflate our numbers!

Counted like that, we take out the 5 variations that occur with both feet on the floor, leaving 40 variations. Then we *double* that number (40 for the left and 40 for the right), producing a total of *80 variations* of the non-symmetrical positions. Then we add back the 5 variations when both feet are on the floor, for a whopping total of *85 possible variations* in your sitting position—if you count that way.

In theory, you really do have that many potential sitting positions! But in practice, people rarely sit with total flexibility on each side. Generally, one side will be favored over the other. So "45" (40 + 5) is closer to the number of variations that any one individual will actually use.

Both Feet on the Floor (1 position, 5 variations)

Sitting with both feet on the floor is pretty close to sitting in a chair. Changing the position of the feet takes you progressively closer to cross-legged sitting, but whichever way you sit, it's a fine position for meditation.

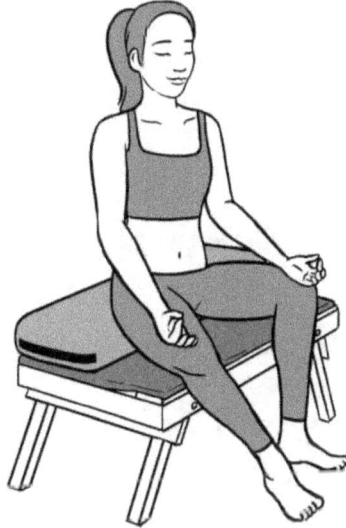

This progression starts from a position that is pretty much like sitting in a chair, and takes you closer to sitting with one or both feet on the bench.

1.   Feet flat on the floor, in line with the thighs

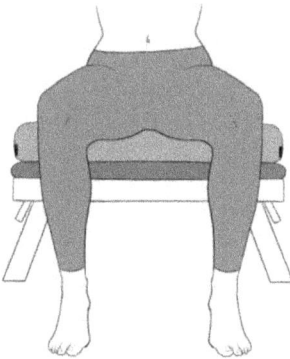

2. Feet pulled in, heels touching, still flat on the floor

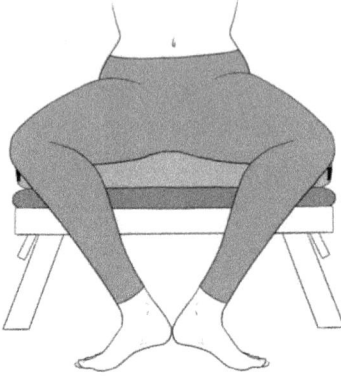

3. One foot pulled in further, with feet crossed

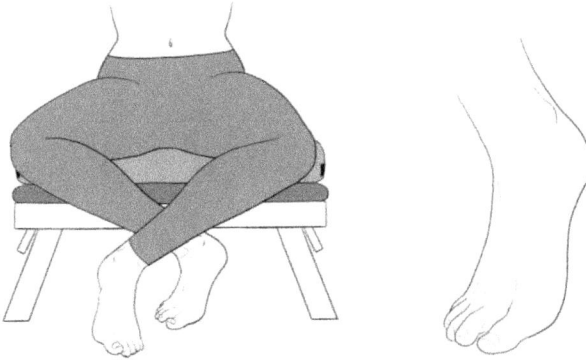

- Weight on the ball of the foot, heel slightly lifted
- The other leg crosses in back, calf cradled in the heel

4. Feet crossed, with edges of feet on the floor

- With your feet out in front of you, you can angle your leg so the edge of the foot is on the floor, like the one shown here:

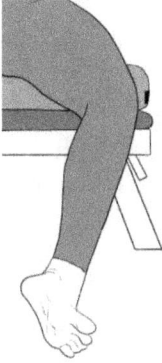

- You can then cross the other ankle over it.
- In that relaxed position, the edges of one or both feet are on the floor.

5. Lower foot turned so top of foot is on the floor, feet crossed

- You can also pull your lower foot back and tuck it under the bench, so the weight is on the outside part of the top of the foot and small toes, as shown here:

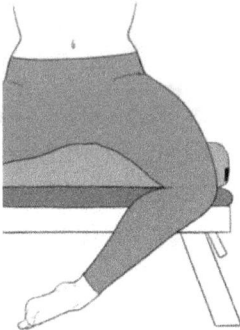

- The other leg crosses in back of that foot, cradled in the heel.
- This is a fairly strenuous position, however, rarely used.

One Foot On the Bench (2 positions, 17 variations for each leg, 34 total)

Many people find that sitting with one foot on the bench and one on the floor is the ideal way to put their back into the perfect upright position for meditation. That position encourages a tilt of the position that centers your spine over the middle of the tripod created by your thighs and the space between your knees.

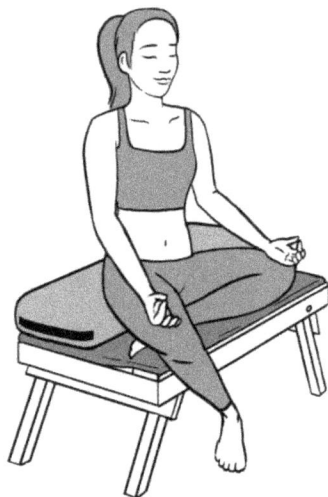

It's possible to achieve that pelvic tilt when sitting in a chair, but a chair doesn't encourage it. And it's possible to do it when sitting with both legs crossed, but for most, a lack of flexibility prevents it. Sitting on the seat cushion with one foot up on the bench seems to induce that position naturally—especially in men.

> *Note:*
> Bringing the thigh of your upper closer to the center of your body tends to reduce pressure on the knee. Moving the knee more to the side tends to increase the pressure while taking you closer to a cross-legged sitting position.

Foot Variations

For the foot on the floor, there is a progression of positions. Each position in the progression takes you closer to a cross-legged position with that leg, with the thigh rotated more to the outside, the lower leg rotated more, and the knee lowered more until ultimately it rests on the bench:

1. Foot flat on the floor, in line with the thigh.

   - The same as sitting in a chair.

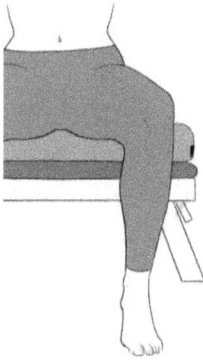

2. Foot pulled in, heel in and toe out, still flat on the floor.

   - The same as sitting with heels together when both feet are on the floor.

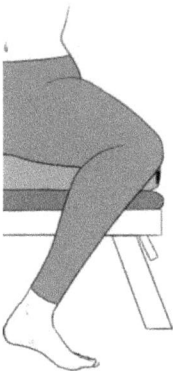

3. Foot pulled in further, on ball of foot, heel raised.

    - The ball of the foot comes closer to the centerline of the body, which   raises   the   heel   farther   off   the   ground.

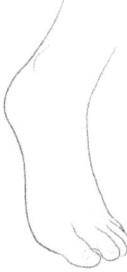

4. Lower leg extended, on edge of foot.

    - Your foot is where it would be when sitting as though in a chair, but this time it's rotated so it is resting on the outer edge of the foot.

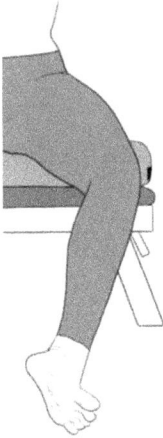

5. Foot pulled in, on edge of foot.
    - Foot is pulled back to center and rotated outward.
    - Ankle is bent. Outside edge of foot is on the ground.
    - Weight will tend to be on the outside edge of the ball of the foot. Heel tends to be unweighted or even slightly raised.

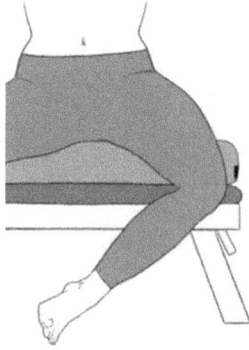

6. Foot pulled in, weight on top of outer toes.

    •   Ankle is straightened. Lower leg is rotated more.

    •   Foot rests on the tops of the small toes and the area of the foot just behind them.

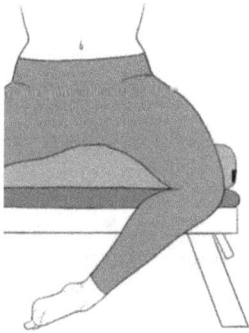

Leg Variations

Sitting with one foot up gives you so many possible variations! To start with, you can put the other foot on the bench with knee raised. That position minimizes the tilt of your pelvis and minimizes pressure on the knee that is working its way towards the bench, getting closer as you relax and as you get more flexible.

From there, you bring the knee progressively lower with one of three positions for the upper leg. Each position in the progression lowers the knee a little more, increasing the tilt of the pelvis, which improves your posture. (But it can also increase pressure on the knee.)

1. **Thigh over the shin**.

    In this position, the thigh is angled slightly beyond the centerline of the body, towards the opposite knee.

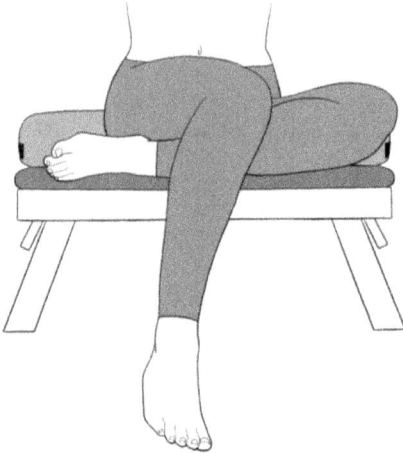

    The position is similar to the Half Tailor pose described later. The difference is that the thigh on the bench is angled comfortably out to the side, instead of tucked in towards the centerline of the body.

2. **Thigh over the heel**.

    This is an intermediate position. Here, the thigh goes straight forward over the upper heel.

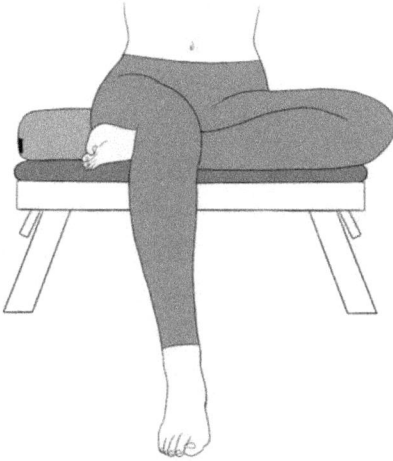

3. **Thigh outside the heel, resting in the arch of the foot.**
    This position is where you want your upper leg to be, ideally.
    It comes very close to sitting cross-legged. The thigh is now
    angled outward, away from the body's centerline. The thigh
    is now cradled in the arch, between the thigh and ball of the
    foot, in a close approximation of cross-legged sitting.

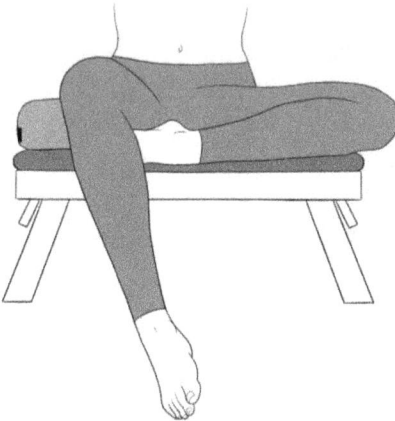

Each position brings the knee slightly lower, increasing the tilt of the
pelvis and the pressure on the lower leg. And for each, the amount of
pressure can be micro-adjusted using the foot-positions described in the
previous section.

Each leg position can be further varied by changing the position of the lower foot. The position of the leg position makes a big change. The position of the foot makes a more minor one. Together, they create a sequence of micro-changes you can use both to get comfortable, and to make progress.

At the extreme, with the thigh outside the heel and the foot pulled in fully, the pelvis is tilted to the maximum extent possible, which brings the back perfectly upright—but when both knees are resting on the bench, there is no *feeling* of pressure.

Half Tibetan (12 variations for each leg, 24 total)

In the full Tibetan Pose (also known as Burmese Pose), both legs are crossed, but one foot is in front of the other. That position is similar to the standard "Easy Pose", but it eliminates pressure on the ankle and shin of the lower leg. So, when hip and leg flexibility allows it, Tibetan Pose tends to be more comfortable than Easy Pose.

When one foot is on the bench, I call that position the "Half Tibetan" because it too eliminates all pressure on the ankle and shin. This tends to be one of the easiest and best poses for meditation.

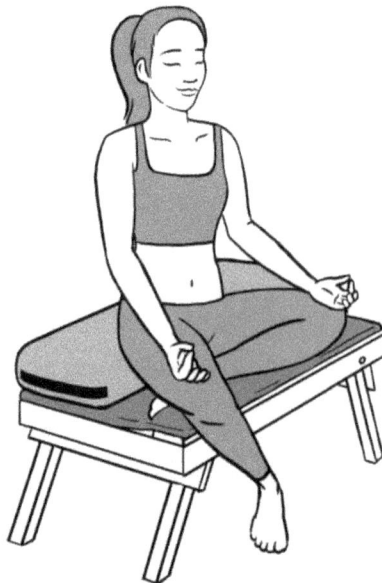

In the Half Tibetan position, the lower foot (on the floor) is in one of the 6 positions above. The upper foot (on the bench) is in one of the 2 positions shown below, creating a total of 6 x 2, or 12 variations.

1. **Half Tibetan pose with bent ankle**
   Like one half of the Easy Pose.

2. **Half Tibetan pose with straight ankle**
   As in the drawing above. A near-perfect position for meditation.

Quarter Lotus (5 variations for each leg, 10 total)

When the upper foot is on your thigh, and the lower foot is on the ground, I call that the *Quarter Lotus Pose* (1/2 of the Half Lotus).

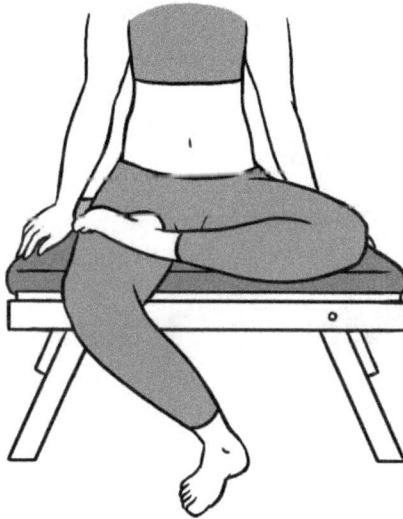

If the upper knee doesn't reach the bench, you can relieve any pressure you may be feeling on the knee in one of several ways:

○   **Angle the seat cushion**, so part of it is under your upper thigh. The extra support for the thigh reduces pressure on the knee.

○   Put **a small cushion** under your thigh for support, as shown on the next page.

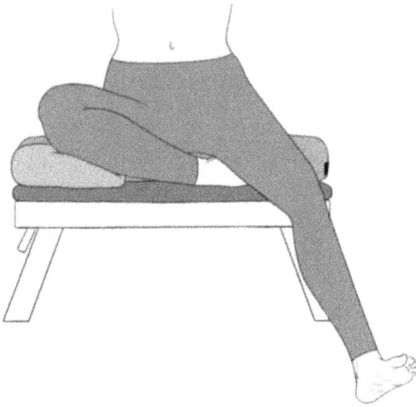

o   Put **a Yoga Block** under your thigh.
    When the block is tilted, it's quite stable—as long as it is on a
    cushion or Yoga Mat and, since your leg is leaning against a flat
    surface, it's really quite comfortable!

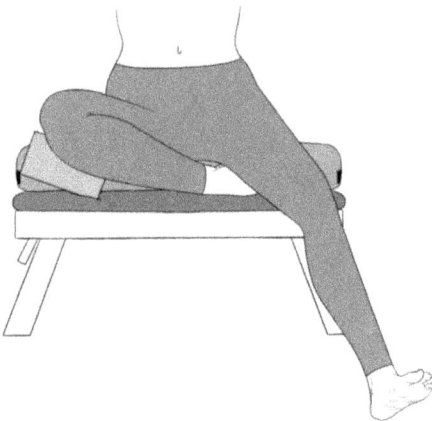

That position is mostly used for the bending asanas that help you move
toward Lotus pose, but it can also be used as a sitting position of its own.

In theory, you have all 6 foot positions for the foot on the floor, but in
practice there is one that gets uncomfortable—when the foot is flat on the
ground, in line with the thigh.

Although that position is certainly possible, the top of the foot presses
down on the thigh bone, and one or the other tends to get uncomfortable
quickly. So that is not a variation you're likely to use.

The other 5 variations have your lower foot pulled inward, toward the center line of your body. In that position the upper leg rotates, exposing the inner thigh. The foot then rests on the fleshy part of the inner thigh, which is a lot more comfortable for most.

One Knee Raised (2 positions, 12 variations for each leg, 24 total)

Varying your sitting position helps to keep you comfortable when sitting for an extended period of time. The position of the lower leg creates the variations. (There are also several variations in the positions of your hands. Those are discussed in a later section.)

Easy Knee Position (7 variations for each leg, 14 total)

Putting one foot flat on the bench and raising the knee so it is at the level of the chin is one way to mix things up a bit. It isn't recommended for meditation or asanas, particularly, but it provides variety when listening to a talk or watching a video.

It's also a great warm-up position. When one of my legs is being stiff, and the knee doesn't want to make it all the way down to the bench, this is a great way to get it to relax enough to get there.

The variations are:

1. Other foot on the floor, in one of the 5 positions described earlier (5 variations).

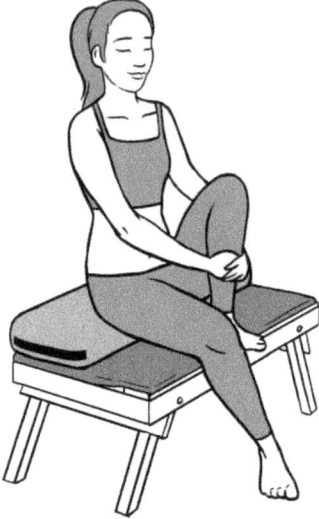

2. Other leg extended, which lets you use it as a counter-balance as you lean back or rock back and forth.

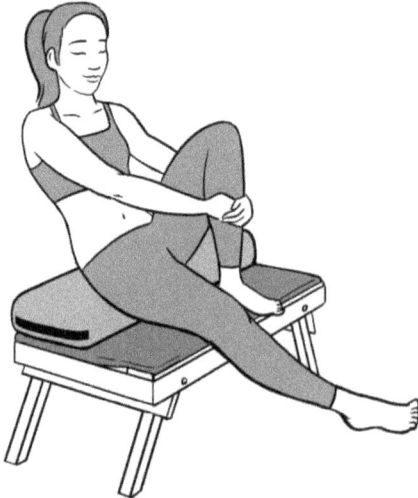

3.   Other foot on the bench, tucked behind the raised knee.

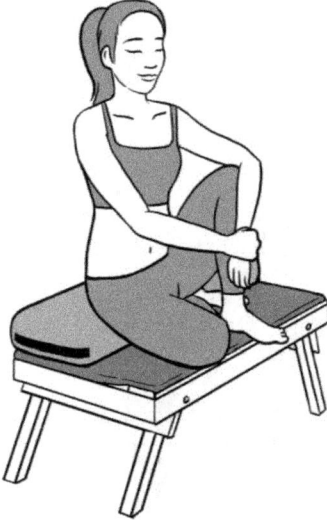

- The foot on the bench has the ankle straight or bent (2 variations).

- You can still rock back and forth in this position, although not quite as much.

- Rocking back even a little does a lot to reduce the pressure on your leg. That's what makes this position such a great warmup for a stiff leg.

- When the leg is warmed up enough that you can come forward with your foot resting on the bench, instead of hovering over it, you can put that foot on the floor to increase pressure slightly on the tucked-in leg, or you can put that foot on top of the tucked-in leg to increase it pressure on it by a lot.

Note:
The "rocking" version can be particularly pleasant. It's like sitting in a rocking chair, and it hearkens back to the kind of rocking we enjoyed as babies and small children. It's relaxing, and probably as good for the brain now, when we're older, as it was when we were young! (We'll have more to say on that subject later on.)

Half Tailor (5 variations for each leg, 10 total)

In this position, the foot on the bench is wrapped around you to the other side of your body, which brings the knee close to the centerline of your body.

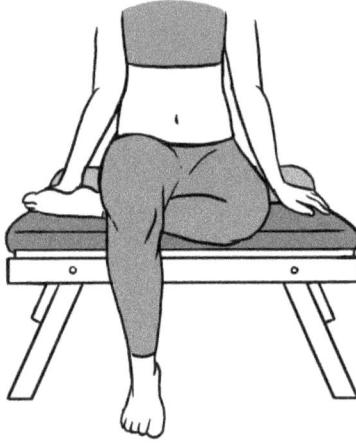

The full position, sitting on the ground, used to be called *Tailor Pose,* because old time tailors in India used to sit that way to sew. (The 5 variations are created by the foot on the floor.)

These days, the full pose would best be known as *Gomukhasana*—cow face pose. But I still like the name *Tailor Pose*, for a couple of reasons.

One reason is that it is the first name I learned for this position, from a wonderful, short, inspiring book that got me started in Yoga back when stones were young: The Yoga System of Health and Relief from Tension, by Yogi Vithaldis. (Short, but detailed. And inspiring.)

The other reason is that in a documentary called Gandhi's Awakening, a little beyond five minutes in, there is a scene of Gandhi sitting on a bench with one foot down and other foot up in that position. He appears to be working with others to make thread or yarn from cotton.

As he sits on the bench, one foot is resting on the floor, the other is wrapped around to his other side. Awesome! The perfect picture of the Half Tailor pose. A web search revealed a still pic of the same pose:

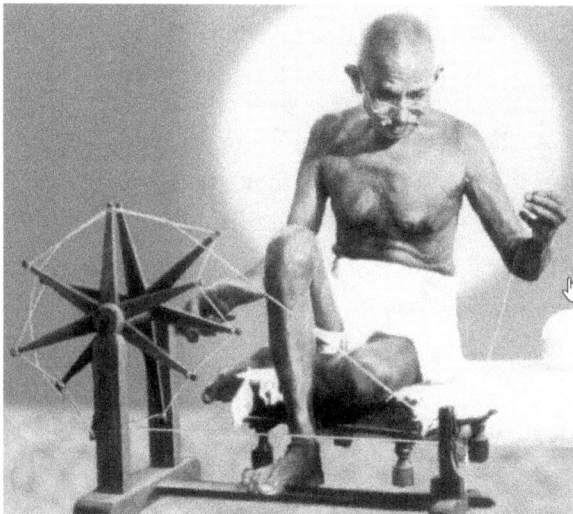

If you do the pose well, your upper thigh will be resting on the lower one, and your upper foot will be resting on its outer edge.

If you do it less well (I'm an expert on this position), your upper foot will be nearly flat on the bench, and your knee will be sticking up in the air—much like the Easy Knee Position. The foot may not even make it all the way down to the bench!

In either of the less-than-truly-adept versions, you'll wind up grasping your shin to pull yourself forward into a more upright position. So it becomes *very much* like the Easy Knee Position, but with the foot in a different place on the bench. You can even rock a bit!

Both Feet on the Bench (6 positions, 11 variations, 22 total)

In Lotus Pose, there is only position for each foot. For the other sitting positions, the foot closest to the foot rail is in one of one of the two positions described above (ankle bent or ankle straight).

The position of the top foot creates one of the other 5 "standard" cross-legged poses shown below, for a total of 10 variations. (Plus Lotus makes 11.)

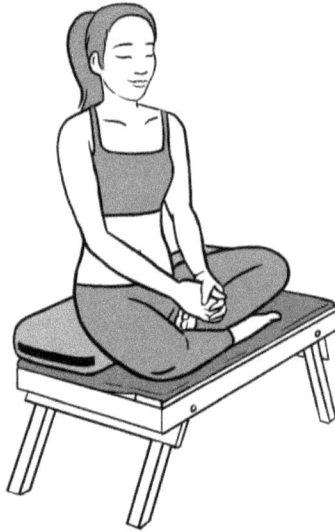

The remainder of this section describes the possible positions. Doing left and right versions of each position creates a total of 22 variations.

Easy Pose

In this position, one leg crosses over the other, and each foot is under the other leg. Here is what you see when you look down at your feet:

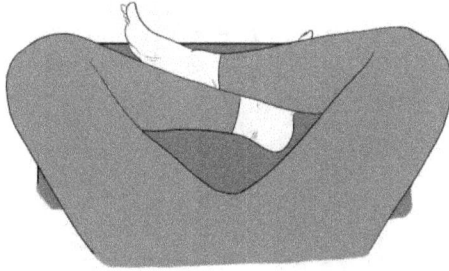

Although this position is easy to get into, when done on the floor it tends to quickly produce pain in the shins and ankles. The various forms of pressure it induces also tend to shut off the nerves, which causes the feet to fall asleep.

The bench makes the position much more comfortable, primarily because of the action of the foot rail. But even so, there are some useful positioning tips that can make it even more comfortable.

The primary tip is that the calf of one leg is cradled by the arch of the other foot, or rests on the ball of the foot. The calf of the other leg, meanwhile, is cradled by the hollow between the ankle bone and heel of the foot it is resting on.

That position minimizes pressure, pain, and prevents the pins-and-needles sensation that occurs when a sleeping leg wakes up.

Tibetan Pose

In this position, one leg crosses *in front* of the other, rather than *over* it.

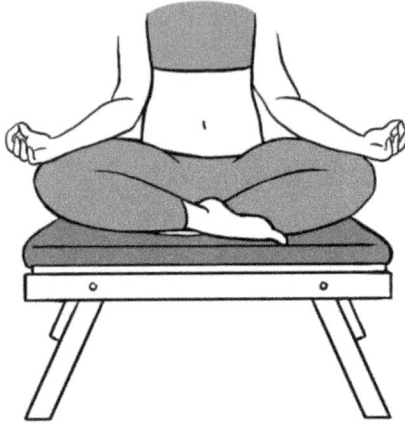

For the inner foot, the heel rests against the other thigh. In fact, the arch of the foot can cradle the thigh. For the outer foot, the heel rests against the other shin.

Here's what you see when looking down at your feet:

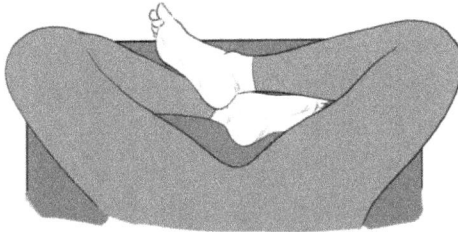

The position is easier when your ankles are in close proximity to one another. When they are far apart, more flexibility is needed in the hips and groin.

The position is most easily adopted when sitting at the desired 15-degree angle, as when sitting on a cushion, either on the bench or on the floor.

Perfect Pose

In Perfect Pose, also called "Meditative Pose of the Adept" by Yogi Vithaldis, both legs are crossed with one foot resting on the other calf.

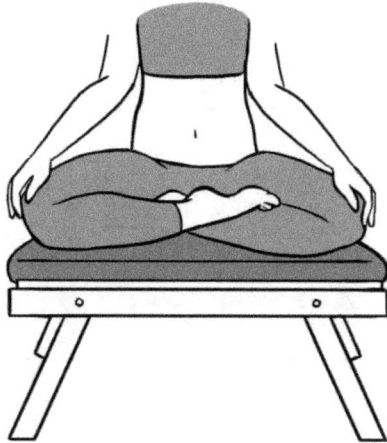

It's a comfortable position—the next step up from Tibetan Pose, and one that begins to move you towards Half Lotus.

Here's what you see when looking down at your feet:

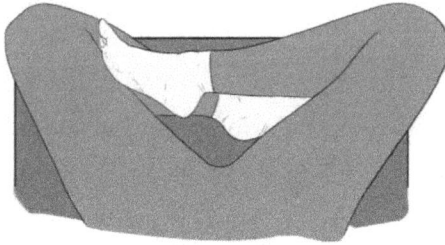

Half Lotus

In Half Lotus, both legs are crossed, with the upper foot on the opposite thigh. It requires more flexibility in the ankles and hips, but it is very stable, which makes it great for meditation.

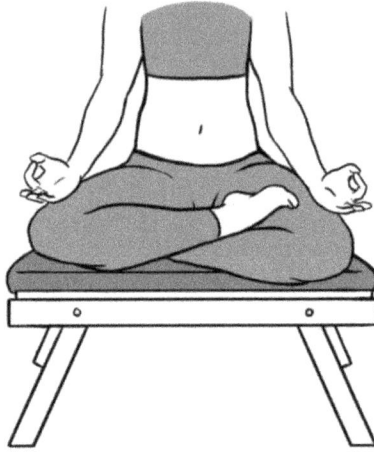

In this position, the upper thigh rests in the arch of the lower foot. (Or, more accurately, it is supported by the heel and ball of the foot.)

The key is this: If you're feeling pain in your knees or strain in your ankles, then it is your *hips* that need opening. Work on the sitting position asanas to do that.

The reason is that your hip flexibility is what allows your thigh to rotate outward. If it rotates easily enough, the knee comes down to the bench without having to force it.

In combination with that rotation, the lower leg *also* rotates outward ("forward", when it is crossed in front of you). That rotation minimizes the bending in the ankle.

Without the required rotations, there is extra pressure on the ankle joint, or a "pinching" sensation at the inner corner of the knees—which forces you keep your knee up to minimize the strain. Or perhaps the knee simply can't go down far enough to get comfortable.

By doing the sitting asanas regularly, and by sitting for longer periods of time (5-10 minutes) in easier poses, you will rapidly develop the ability to get into this position.

Tailor Pose

In Tailor Pose, one knee is in front, with the foot wrapping around to the other side of your body. The other leg crosses *over* that one and wraps around to the side as well.

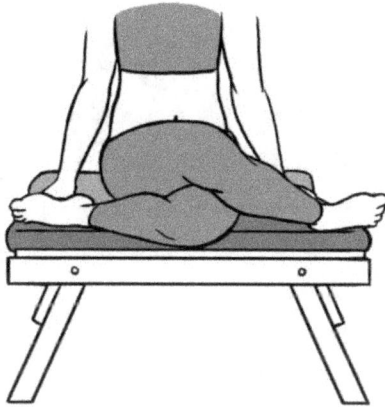

I confess that I do not find this position comfortable. At all. I lack the flexibility to do it properly—which means I clearly need to do it more! (At the very least, I need to make sure I have Half Tailor in my sitting-position rotation.)

Done well, your upper thigh rests on the lower one, and your upper foot rests on its outer edge. Done less well, you do what you can to get your upper foot to the bench, and try to minimize the degree to which the knee sticks up in the air.

Lotus Pose

This position is much more accurately called "Pretzel Pose". The idea is that the legs wrap over each other, and each foot winds up on the opposite thigh.

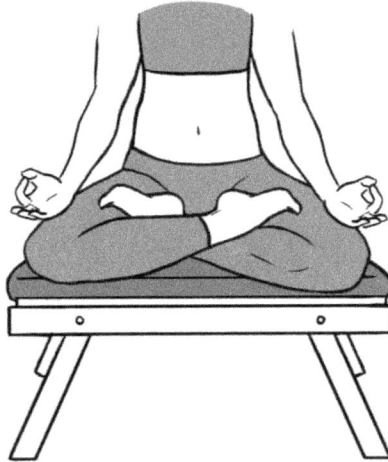

It's a great position for meditation—when you can sit in it *comfortably*. If it's *not* comfortable, don't force yourself into it. That produces injury.

Lots of great meditations happen in Half Lotus—or any other position you can comfortably hold, so focus your attention there, unless you find Lotus easy to get into, and easy to stay in.

If you can sit in Half Lotus comfortably for 20 minutes, *on each side*, then you are probably ready to give Lotus Pose a try.

Intermediate Positions

These intermediate positions could easily be considered as unique positions in their own right. But there are many positions, with small variances between them, so it makes more sense to consider them separately.

Yoga Block Footstool

You've gone through the 5 foot-position progressions to prepare for putting one foot up on the bench. But you still can't quite manage it,

Or maybe you have one foot up, but can't quite get the other foot up on the bench, even in one of the easier positions.

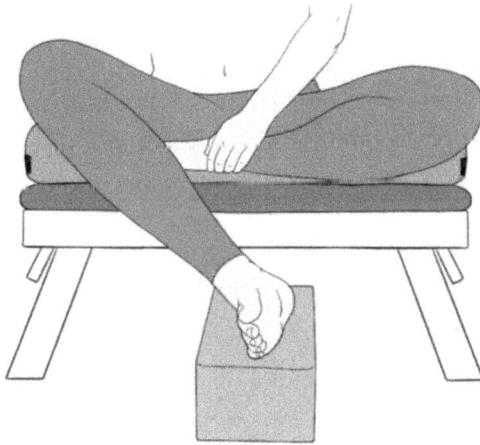

In situations like that, you can use a Yoga Block as a footstool! Put it on the floor in front of you in one of its three orientations (high, medium, or low), and rest your lower foot or ankle on it!

Tip:
If the block is on a mat or soft carpet, you can let it tip a bit as you put your foot on it. Because of the cushioned surface it's resting on, it won't tip over or slide away--and it will be at exactly the angle you need to support your leg or foot.

Hand Holding Foot

Let's say you're in Half Tibetan pose, with one foot up on the bench. The next big step is Quarter Lotus, with your foot on your outer thigh. The only problem is, that's a pretty big jump!

Sitting in Half Tibetan, your muscles have warmed up and your flexibility has improved, but it's still a long way from there to Half Lotus. What do you do?

The answer is an intermediate position. If your left foot is on the bench, grasp the edge of your foot with your right hand and rest your hand against the side of your thigh.

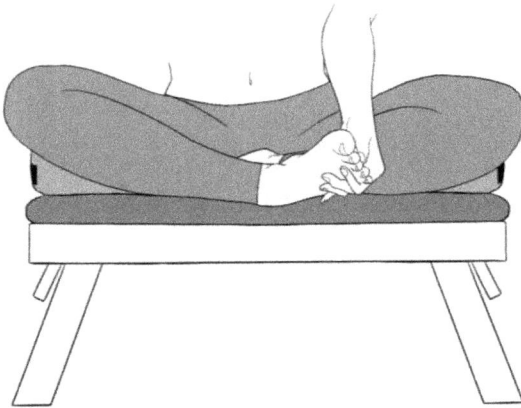

Depending on where you rest your hand, you can hold the foot closer to the Half Tibetan position, or closer to the Quarter Lotus position. In other words, you can use your hand to create a variety of intermediate positions. It's a way to get there from here!

The bending asanas discussed later are more difficult to do in these positions (although not impossible), but for just sitting and relaxing, holding a foot with one hand is hard to beat.

You can do the same thing when sitting with both legs up.

Combination Easy Pose & Tibetan Pose

In Easy Pose, each leg is crossed over the other foot. In Tibetan Pose, each of the lower legs is rotated so that neither one is over the other foot.

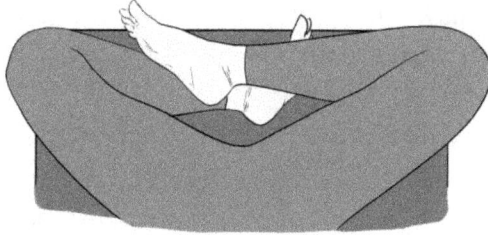

In the combination pose, the inner ankle is bent, so the outer leg rests on the ball of the inner foot. But the outer ankle is straight, with the heel angled *against* the inner calf, rather than supporting it.

This combination of Easy Pose and Tibetan Pose could easily be considered as a unique new position, all its own. But I prefer to think of it as "transition" pose that helps you take the next step from Easy Pose.

Hand Positions

In terms of "internal energy flow", much is made of the need to "complete the energy circuit" by joining your hands together, or joining energy centers in the hands to energy centers in the lower body.

I'm not sure I buy any of that, personally. Of course, I have to leave open the possibility that it makes a significant difference, and I am just not aware of it as yet. But it is equally possible the difference is so subtle that it's like putting a coat of wax on a car.

If I'm right about that, then getting the legs oriented comfortably is like getting the frame aligned in the car, getting the back centered over that tripod is like getting the engine working properly, and getting your hands into a comfortable position is like getting the body of the car set up, so it keeps out the wind and the rain as you drive.

If so, then the final energetic connection of the hands is the finishing touch—like a shiny coat of wax. So if your body is the vehicle that takes you down the path towards enlightenment, then creating a strong sitting posture is the way you get the car running smoothly.

However, so *much* is made of "completing the circuit" in both Yoga and Oriental internal energy traditions like Taiji and Chi Gong, that I am forced to admit that there may be elements of the practice that I do not yet perceive and understand.

In short, take what follows as a guide to help you choose hand positions that work for you. Then apply whatever "circuit connection" strategy your local guru suggests.

As you'll see, different hand positions make it easier or harder to get your back aligned properly. If your guru demands a hand position that is incompatible with what you need to achieve that alignment, then it may be time to find a new guru—or work harder to achieve a better sitting position, so that the guru's hand position works for you.

Finally, it is important to note that all of the hand positions have one thing in common: The arms are *fully relaxed*, with the *elbows hanging below the shoulders.*

> ***Whichever hand position you use,***
> ***the arms are fully relaxed,***
> ***with the elbows hanging below the shoulders.***

Hands Cupped in Lap

When your hands are in your lap, you can cup them, so the back of one hand sits in the palm of the other. Thumbs can be touching at the tips as shown here, or they can lie next to one another.

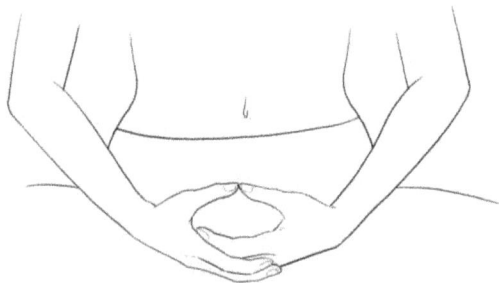

When your hands are cupped, Yoga systems and Oriental internal energy systems both suggest that the thumbs should be lightly touching, to "complete the energy circuit". I don't personally know that it makes any difference, but why not do it? If nothing else, it shows that you are one of the cool kids.

The most important thing to know about having your hands in your lap is that it is a great way to *test* your sitting position.

With your hands in your lap, you can't use your arms to pull your back into an upright, balanced position. So if you can sit comfortably with your hands in your lap, it means that your sitting position is perfect—no assistance is required from your arms.

If you find it hard to sit comfortably in that manner, consider using one of the other hand positions. As we go through the list of options, you'll find that they make it progressively easier to pull your back into an upright posture that is centered over your leg-tripod.

Yoga Interlace in Lap

You can also *interlace* your fingers while holding your hands in your lap.

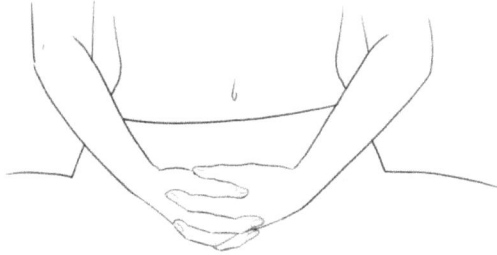

When you do, interlace them *Yoga-style*, with the little fingers overlapping one other, instead of crossing over each other. Overlapped, they create a smooth surface for positions like headstand, so there is no pressure on the bottom pinkie finger.

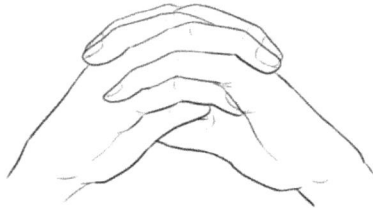

Hands on Knees, Palms Up

In this position, your palm is facing "upward". It's not facing up, exactly, and it's not facing to the side. It's an angle between those two.

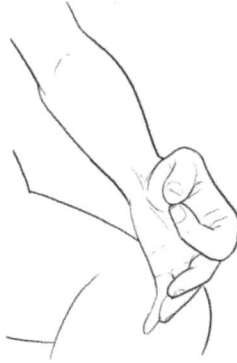

This position is one of my favorites, because it also lets you exert a subtle pull with your hands that helps to get your back into position, with your head centered over your leg-tripod.

When all you need is a small, subtle assist, this is a great position to use, because even a subtle pull helps tilt your pelvis and arch your lower back into the "J curve" that positions your head and upper back over the center of your leg-tripod.

The other cool thing about this hand position is that the edge of the hand fits nicely into the small curve between the knee bones—a curvature that is exposed when the knees are down and to the sides, relative to the hips.

To "complete the energy circuit" in this position, the tip of your index fingers lightly touch the tips of your thumbs. That position is known as *Yoga Mudra*—the symbol of Yoga.

Hands on Knees, Palms Down

This position lets you use your arms to exert a strong pull—one that is pretty much guaranteed to pull your back into alignment.

The traditions that insist on completing an energy circuit would never recommend this position, or the ones that follow. But I like to think that the energy centers in the palms of the hands are connected to the energy centers in the ankles.

In any case, "needs must", as they say in Britain. If you *need* to get your back into alignment so you can sit comfortably, it is possible that you *must* use this hand position, or one like it.

Hands on Feet or Ankles

When you're in an intermediate position where one hand is holding your foot, you'll find that you can use that hand to help pull your back forward.

You can pull even more strongly if you put the other hand on your ankle, or use it to cup the foot with both hands, one on top of the other.

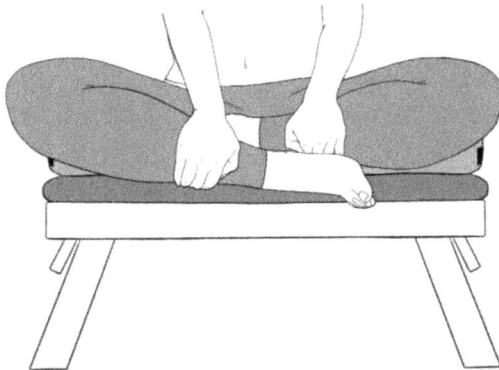

When both legs are crossed, you can also grasp your feet or ankles to pull your back forward. Those positions may violate the "energy circuit" rules, but they can do your back a world of good!

Hands on a Raised Knee

When one foot is flat on the bench with the knee raised, your hands can be in a variety of positions—each of which can help to alleviate strain in your back. In each position, the arms pull against the leg, and the leg pulls against the back, all with the same kind of effort it takes to stand upright—in other words, very little!

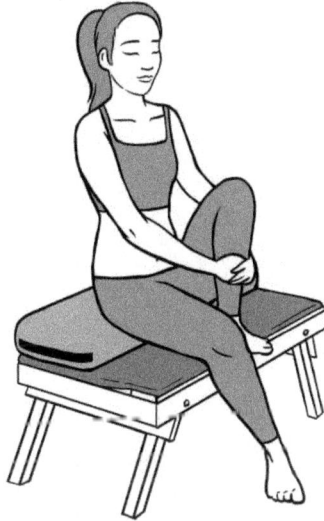

○ **Wrist on shin**

- If your left knee is up, you can wrap your left wrist around the shin, and grasp your left wrist with your right hand.

- In that position, your left hand is loose and relaxed. It's not doing much of anything.

- Your right hand, in the meantime, *also* isn't doing much of anything. The fingers are curled around the wrist, but for some reason that doesn't seem to require any strength.

○ **Elbow on knee, grasping the arm**

- If your left knee is up, you can wrap your left arm around it so the knee is sitting in the crook of your elbow.

- In that position, the left arm hangs down, while the right hand curls around the left forearm or wrist.

○ **Elbow on knee, arms folded**

- Your left elbow curls around the knee, as before, but this time the left hand comes back towards your right shoulder.

- It may make it all the way to your shoulder, or it may wind up resting on the right bicep. Either way, the right hand goes up and over the left forearm, with the fingers curling around the left elbow.

Growing-to-Lotus Sitting Asanas

To my mind, these are the most important asanas you can do, because they help you move towards the Lotus position.

For more than a year, these were pretty much *all* I did. In time, the other exercises and asanas described in this book came to me—at times internally, during the meditative parts of my practices, and at other times as a result of seeing how other asanas and exercises could be adapted to the bench.

So much came to me as a result of sitting in meditation, on the bench, that meditation became pretty much the most important part of the day. As I learned to apply energization techniques, and as I developed into a "strong sitter", the meditations became ever more profound.

So, yes. I highly recommend these asanas. If you do nothing else with the bench, do these.

Why Lotus?

Of course, it is probably worth asking, "What makes Lotus Pose so valuable?" It's a darn good question, and one you should know the answer to, because it is a primary motivation for using the bench to perform these asanas.

Why Do the Sitting Asanas at all?

After all, the bench lets you sit in a variety of ways that are conducive to meditation. Isn't that enough? Why do extra asanas to move towards the Lotus position?

There are several reasons for doing the asanas:

1.   They increase flexibility, making more positions available to you.
2.   They release energy.
3.   They help you get to Lotus Pose, eventually. (Next, we'll talk about *why* you want to do that.)

Why Sit in Lotus Position?

Lotus Pose is highly desirable, for some very good reasons.

> *Important!*
> Here, I am talking about being able to sit in Lotus Position
> *without strain*. If you have to force yourself into position, or
> have to strain to stay there, you risk injury, and will most
> likely do yourself more harm than good. So take it easy, and
> go to Lotus position *when you're ready* to get there.

You want to be able to sit in Lotus Position, if you can, for several
reasons. For one thing, if you can sit in Lotus, you don't really need a
cushion. The bench helps to make that point clear. When you can sit in
Quarter Lotus, with one foot in Half Lotus and the other the floor, it
becomes evident that sitting on a cushion isn't any more comfortable than
sitting directly on the bench. In fact, in some ways it is *less* comfortable.

With your foot in Quarter Lotus position, the knee is farther away from
the bench, so it's easier to get it to a resting position without the cushion.
And while the cushion helps to keep pressure off of your feet in easier
poses, it doesn't make any difference in full Lotus. So for knee support and
foot comfort, the cushion is unnecessary. That just leaves the pelvic tilt that
puts your back in its most comfortable upright position.

In Lotus Pose, I estimate that the cushion doesn't even do that much for
the tilt of the pelvis! I'm forced to extrapolate here, because only one of my
legs (having had fewer surgeries) is flexible enough to get into Lotus
position. But with that leg in position, I don't see the big increase in my
pelvic tilt, the way I do when the leg is in Half Tibetan position, for
instance.

The reason is that, when your foot is on your thigh, the pelvis can only
tilt so far! So Lotus pose may help to keep you from *over*-arching your
back. In other words, it might just make it easier to find the point of perfect
balance.

So one reason for wanting to sit in Lotus is that you can dispense with
the cushion. Another is that it may help you achieve a perfectly balanced,
perfectly upright spine.

But there are other important reasons for wanting to sit in Lotus that may be even more important:

1. You basically cannot fall over.

2. *Because* you can't fall over, at the point where you start to fall asleep, you are woken up by a slight nod of the head, rather than by falling to the side.

That last bit is important because, if your body falls over, it produces an *adrenaline response* that takes you right out of your relaxed, meditative state.

At the same time, you want to be so fully relaxed that you are at the *threshold* of sleep. That threshold is known as the alpha/theta crossover.

Alpha/Theta Crossover

When you're in the *alpha* state, you're relaxed and aware. In the *theta* state, you're sleeping.

In the *deep alpha* state, you're extremely relaxed, and very close to sleeping. When you cross over into *light theta*, you begin to dream as you access images and sensations that are beyond (or below) your conscious awareness.

When you are in deep meditation, you're not on one side of the boundary or the other. Instead, you *dip down* into theta for a bit, then *rise up* into alpha, and repeat the cycle.

That's known as the *Alpha/Theta Crossover* state.

That state is important, because you are interacting directly with your subconscious mind. In that state, subconscious memories can surface and rise into conscious awareness.

Thoughts, suggestions, ideas, and affirmations can go the other way, as well. In that state, your affirmations bypass your conscious filters and go directly into your subconscious, where they are perceived as *truth*—an internal understanding that is integrated into your being, which no conscious logic can touch.

That state is the foundation for hypnotism, affirmation therapy, lucid dreaming, sleep learning, and Yoga Nidra (a near-sleep affirmation process). It's what makes those practices work. In that state, you are in touch with deep emotional memories that dominate our thinking and decision-making processes, in ways we generally neither recognize nor understand. It is a time when you can access those memories, and (if you want) change the self-perceptions and decisions that are based on them.

That state is also the basis of really *deep* meditation. Other sitting positions help to pave the way. They let you meditate well enough to make a huge difference in your life. But to go really deep, you need Lotus Pose.

> *Note:*
> It is worth repeating that here, I am talking about a Lotus Position that you can assume *easily*, and maintain *comfortably*. Anything else produces injury that *harms* your vehicle. It's like getting a flat tire on a remote road—except you don't have a spare! You want a strong vehicle that will carry you *comfortably* on your journey to enlightenment. So take it easy!

The Dynamic "Subtle Energy" Sequence

Now that we know *why* we want to do the sitting asanas, let's talk about *how* to do them—and how to make other asanas more effective, as well.

> *Note:*
> The sequence of movements described in this section works like *magic* for forward bends—and those are *key* to improving your sitting flexibility.

Have Yoga Block(s) Ready

When you're doing an asana or pose that you want to spend some time in, it's helpful to have a Yoga Block on hand, for support.

To make things even easier, have two Yoga Blocks. (I keep one on each side of my bench.)

Having one block in each hand makes it easy to work your way down to progressively lower positions and (perhaps more importantly!) work your way back up again.

Breathe into Position to Start

To get started, get into position and breathe. Try to relax a little further each time you exhale, but don't push yourself. A millimeter or two may be what is available to you at this stage. If so, that's fine.

On the other hand, perhaps you're just a little stiff. In that case, you wind up moving several inches as you relax, or even more. That's great, too.

The point is just to breathe in, then exhale and relax. As you inhale, it can help to pull back just slightly. For example, in a forward bend, you can lift your head and straighten your back a little, then let your head fall and round your back as you exhale.

The point is to relax. Feel your body. Find what works. Loosen up, and let go.

The Power of Rocking

You don't necessarily have to do any more than just sit in a given position. If you just "hang out" there for a while, your body automatically relaxes and adjusts to it, so it becomes easier. Eventually, you'll be ready for the next stage.

A small amount of rocking can make it that much better.

Back during my martial arts training, I used to find that my torso was engaged in a small back-forth-movement as I was meditating. That small movement is called *rocking*.

Later, I would find that it is a sign of internal energy flowing. All I knew for sure was that I was "away" for a while (gone to wherever you go during deep meditation), my body did the rocking all on its own so that when I came back, I found the rocking going on.

I stress that it is a small, subtle movement. When I became aware of it, I could increase it as much as I wanted. But to the degree I could let go and just let it happen on its own, it was a very small movement.

During my Raja Yoga training, instructor Tandava related that, in the Jewish tradition, it's called "Davening". Apparently someone saw David doing it and thought, "He's an enlightened soul, and he does it. Maybe I should do it, too."

Whereupon everyone started doing it. So there are people who rock back and forth as hard they can—mostly during prayer, but I have seen it during a computer class, as well. Apparently, the idea is that vigorous rocking will bring them closer to God.

Who knows? Maybe it does! Or maybe it just keeps you more alert. Or maybe it just feels good. However, in my experience the small subtle movement the body does on its own—without conscious assistance—is sufficient. And it can have strong physical and mental effects.

Physically, the rocking movement puts a slight amount of pressure on the pelvis and legs (depending on how you're sitting), followed by an immediate relaxation of that pressure. So it's kind of like doing a Yoga pose for a micro-second, and then immediately following it with Savasana (the relaxing pose) for another micro-second.

Physically, then, rocking is a great way to increase flexibility.

> *Note:*
> You should know that, when doing Yoga, your flexibility is generally going to increase at the rate of about a millimeter a day—or a fraction thereof. In other words, while you can expect steady, constant progress, it's best not to be in any kind of hurry! One reason rocking is so effective, in all probability, is that it is working right at that edge, to precisely the degree that growth can occur.

Rocking has potentially strong mental effects, too. Studies have shown increased brain development in babies who are rocked by their caregivers.

That growth probably results from the increased visual adjusting needed to make sense of the world, but as children we loved swings, teeter-totters, and other forms of movement. And as adults there is something just wonderfully comforting about a rocking chair. So it is entirely possible that the slight movement of the head produces other beneficial effects that we have yet to fully recognize.

As Health Benefits of Rocking Chairs reports,

> "Rocking is relaxing. It releases endorphins in the brain that improve mood while reducing stress and pain."

For those reasons, rocking also fosters deeper sleep. It also stimulates the inner ear, which improves balance as it increases emotional and psychological well-being, reducing anxiety and depression. It even burns a few calories!

Note:
The "rocking" concept applies to most other asanas, as well.
But in that context, I call it *pulsing.*

Basic Subtle-Energy Enhancements

These enhancements pack a double punch. In addition to increasing the flexibility of the stretch, they produce a noticeable increase in the internal energy flows you may feel if you meditate between asanas (a practice that is highly recommended, by the way).

Of course, there are times when all you really feel like doing is hanging out for a while, and breathing. And that is just fine. On those days, stay in the "Breathe in the Position" mode, which is both the start and end of the sequence.

But when you're feeling like you want a little more of the secret sauce, try these enhancements:

1. Exhaling Pulse
   - After breathing into position for 4 breaths or so (the more the better), take a deep breath and, as you exhale, pulse forward 4 times.

Note:
You may have a number that works better for you. For me, doing things 4 times seems to work well.

- Take another deep breath, and pulse as you exhale once more.
- This pulsing movement is pretty equivalent of rocking while sitting.
- As with all other entries in this sequence, hang out here and do this one as long as it feels good. Or skip it if it doesn't work for you.

2. Healing Squeeze and Relax

- I learned this move in Ananda's Raja Yoga program. It's an enhancement to Raja Yoga that Yogananda taught for healing. I found that it also works beautifully when done as part of a Yoga asana.

Note:
Ananda calls this action "tense and relax". But I'm reserving the word "tension" for what happens without conscious awareness, and "squeeze" for what you do consciously.

- For one thing, this action puts you in touch with your body— you *feel* where the tension is. For another, it helps to release that tension and promote relaxation, right where you need it!
- To do the movement, feel the part of your body that is under tension. For forward bends, I generally find that tension in the hips. But it can also be in the glutes (backside) or hamstrings. (It's *your* body. It could be somewhere entirely different, on you. Wherever it is, find it and feel it.)
- As you inhale, alternately squeeze and relax the muscles in that area. (I like to squeeze and relax 4 times as I inhale. Again, that's my number. In general, I find 4-6 squeezes works well.)
- As you exhale, release all tension and let go. Let gravity extend your body position.
- Repeat the sequence, squeezing and relaxing several times while inhaling, then exhaling and releasing.

- Alternatively, continue squeezing and relaxing while exhaling, in addition to inhaling. You are then applying the "rocking" motion to the asana.

3. Stay Here or Move On

- Listen to your body. Perhaps it wants to stay here and finish for the day. In that case, Breathe in the Position to end the sequence (below).

- Or maybe it wants to stay here for a bit, breathe into the position, and then move on to the "Advanced Subtle-Energy Enhancements" (next).

- Or maybe it is just eager to skip ahead to the next stage! Of course, you won't know what the Advanced Enhancements are like until after you've done them a time or two. But after that, your body will tell you what it wants.

Advanced Subtle-Energy Enhancements

If you thought the last set of enhancements made a difference, stand back and watch out! These are incredible. Do them if you're inclined, or skip ahead to the ending breaths.

1. Maximum Tension & Forward Reach

- As you inhale, put the muscle under as much tension as you can. Squeeze it with all of your might, until it is quivering and shaking.

- Yogananda called this process *Quiver Healing*. (Later on, you'll learn more about its healing and energizing effects.) I like to do it in time with the breath, but you can also do it in a way that spans several breaths. I'm told he taught it various ways: Squeezing while inhaling, squeezing while exhaling, and squeezing continuously while inhaling and exhaling. Find what works for you.

- As you exhale, release the tension.

- While exhaling, reach forward as far as you can.

- Find something to grab, and hold on. (Ankle, toe, shin, bottom of bench, whatever.)

2. Pull-Back Isometric

   - As you inhale, pull backward against the resistance created by what you're holding.

   - In a forward bend, for example, pulling backward with the back muscles produces a highly-desirable tilt of the pelvis.

   - This physical-exertion-without-movement is called an *isometric*, from *iso*-same and *metric*-distance. (We'll have a lot more to say about them in a later chapter on strengthening exercises.)

3. Push-Forward Isometric

   - As you exhale, push forward against resistance.

   - The resistance could be created by your hand on your shin, or on a Yoga Block, or on the top of the bench.

   - When sitting with your knee straight out in front of you, the resistance can be created by your shoulder pressing on your knee, on a hand placed on the knee, or even on a Yoga Block placed on the knee.

   - Whatever it is, push forward against it as strongly as you can while exhaling, all the while resisting the movement.

4. Pull Forward

   - The interesting thing about the push-forward isometric is that your body automatically relaxed the area you're stretching! It's an automatic response to a muscular exertion.

   - As you continue to hold the foot, shin, or bench you grabbed originally, inhale and pull yourself forward.

   - You'll find that you have now gone quite a bit further— perhaps further than ever before in your life!

5. Relax and breathe

- Congratulations! You've gone through the advanced "super sequence", and have now gone quite a bit further—perhaps further than ever!

- Now it's time to relax—*while staying in the position,* or as near to it as is comfortable. This final relaxation is an important part of the process. Don't overlook it! We'll talk more about it, next.

Breathe in the Position to End

If you've done any of the enhancements, you have now progressed further than when you started. Some days, in fact, you will have progressed further than you ever have in your life! It's now time to "hang out" in that new position, and let your body acclimate to it.

For this part of the practice, I like to hang out for 8 to 12 breaths. As when breathing into position, the key is to relax a little on each exhalation. At this stage, of course, you probably won't go any further when you exhale. (You *shouldn't.*) But you should find yourself becoming more relaxed in your new position. And that is key.

It may be that you need to back off a bit to truly relax. That's fine. Back off as much as you need. You will almost certainly be farther than where you started, and if you can relax there, you're doing well.

Dynamic Asanas

The dynamic movements given in the previous section work extremely well for forward bends. But it is difficult to make them work with other asanas.

It is *possible* to do so. And it's a valuable practice for sitting asanas where you are pushing your knee down, for example. In that situation, you reverse the bending progression so that you are initially resisting an upward movement of the knee, then resisting a downward movement, before finally pushing it downward.

But for asanas where you twist your torso, or your neck, there is very little to be gained from such a progression. The same can be said for most of the back bends, and other asanas where you are already at the edge of the flexibility, with little more to be gained. You will still improve over time, but gradually, as there is very little additional flexibility to be gained in any one sitting—unlike the forward bends, where you can frequently gain several *inches* of flexibility in the course of a few breaths.

For asanas of that kind, the dynamic version is a simple isometric at the end of the pose.

Consider a torso twist, for example. You inhale, put one hand on the opposite knee, the other hand behind you, and twist as you exhale. If you are relaxed and breathing slowly, you'll reach your maximum twist before you run out of breath.

When you get to your maximum twist, use the rest of your exhalation for an isometric/isotonic *contraction*. In other words, contract the muscles that are involved in the twist, exerting as much energy as you can to maximize the movement.

As you do, you will notice that you move farther than you thought you could—and you will be strengthening some muscles in the process!

The same sort of muscle contractions can be applied to Cat/Cow Pose, and other poses. Even Tree Pose can benefit from an *isotonic* contraction, where you simply squeeze the muscle, without working against any particular resistance. It's the fastest way to strengthen the muscles you need for balance.

Bending Positions

At this point, we have covered *why*, and *how*. Now let's talk about *what*—as in, what positions to use:

1. Feet on the floor, knees together or parallel – like sitting in a normal chair.

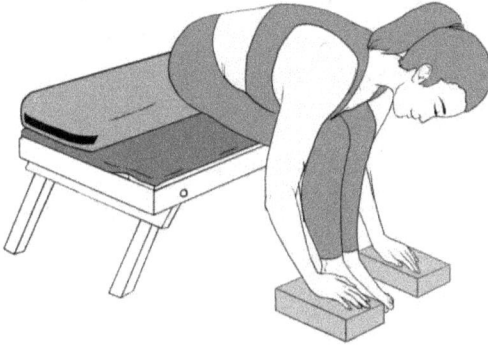

2. **Feet on the floor, knees apart** – like sitting cross-legged, but with feet on floor.

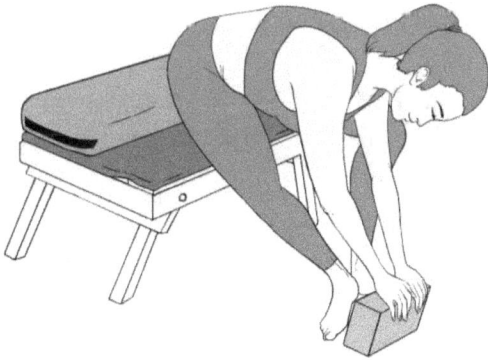

The remaining positions have already been shown. Bend forward in whichever position is comfortable enough to use.

3. **Half Tibetan** – One foot is tucked under your thigh, the other is on the floor.

4. **Quarter Lotus** – One foot is on your thigh, the other is on the floor

5. **Half Lotus** – One foot is on your thigh, the other is on the bench.

Note:

As my Half Lotus position progressed, I noticed a pronounced tendency to slide forward off of my seat cushion. When that starts happening to you, it's time for a smaller cushion! Even better, move forward to the edge of the seat cushion. The edge compresses more easily, so in effect the cushion becomes smaller. Sitting on the edge also makes it easier to achieve the desired tilt of the pelvis. So if you start sliding off the seat cushion, that's a *good* thing. It means you're making progress.

6. **Easy Pose** – Each foot rests under the other leg.

7. **Full Tibetan** – One foot is tucked under your thigh, the other rests in front of it.

8. **Perfect Pose** – One foot is tucked under your thigh. The other rests on your calf.

9. **Lotus Pose** – Also known (perhaps more accurately!) as **Pretzel Position**, with both feet on opposite thighs. Great if you can do it. But *don't force it.*

Reminder:

Any time you have one foot on the floor, you can place that foot on a Yoga Block to make the pose incrementally more difficult.

Movement Patterns

For each sitting asana, do this series of movements.

Knee to the Bench

If your knee is already resting comfortably on the bench, you can skip this movement. Otherwise, continue sitting upright and perform the movement sequence for the knee.

Gently Press on the Knee

With your palm on your knee, gently press the knee towards the bench, as shown in the figure on the next page.

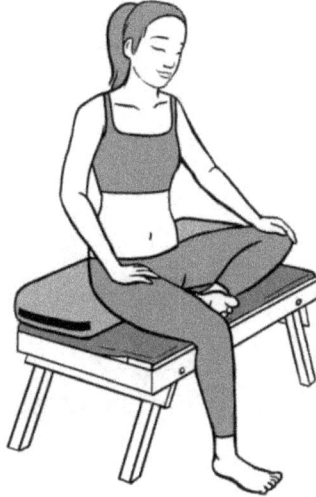

You'll notice that it is easier to do when your lower leg is rotated. That's one of the advantages of working with one foot on the bench. With the other thigh going *over* the foot, it is possible for the ankle to straighten. That straightened ankle makes it easier (or even *possible*) to rotate the lower leg.

Assisted Limb Rotation

That rotation of the lower leg is very important, for advanced sitting positions—for example, Lotus Pose. And it doesn't hurt to rotate the upper leg, as well, because those rotations alleviate the most pain common pain associated with the pose—a pinching sensation at the inner corner of the knee.

Note:
This valuable tip came from Lotus-Pose expert David Keil (*k"eye"-l*) in his YouTube video, Working with the Knee in Lotus.

Keil points out that the most commonly occurring pain in advanced positions is at the inside corners of the knees. To resolve that pain, *rotate the upper and lower legs* away from that point.

Here is what it looks like, looking down at it from above.

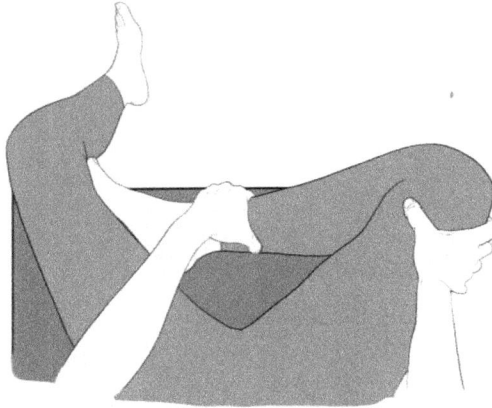

Here is the sequence:

1. Put your outside hand behind your knee.

    - That's your right hand, if right foot is on the bench.
    - Thumb is inside the thigh, behind the knee. Fingers are on the outside of the thigh.
    - Grasp firmly and rotate outward.

2. Put your inside hand on your shin, a little above the ankle.

    - That's your left hand, if right foot is on the bench.
    - Thumb is inside the calf, fingers are outside.
    - Grasp firmly and rotate outward

With the legs rotated as far as possible, allow the leg to fall towards the bench.

If you like, you can also press down gently with the hand near the knee.

This movement does some good things:

○   By removing the pinching sensation, it lets your leg fall to the position that your flexibility *truly* allows.

o   The rotation of the lower leg helps to achieve a comfortable foot position and tilt of the pelvis.

Enhancements

When you have been gently pushing the knee towards the bench for a while (several sessions to develop relaxed flexibility, and enough time in the current session to warm up the leg), you can add these enhancements:

1.   **Pull-Back Isometric**
     Inhaling:

     • Put your hand on top of your knee. Arm is straight.

     • Attempt to pull your knee upward towards your chest, resisting the movement with your arm.

2.   **Push-Forward Isometric**
     Exhaling:

     • Grasp your knee with your hand. Attempt to push your knee down to the bench, resisting the movement with your arm.

3.   **Push Down**
     Inhaling:

     • Use your hand, arm, and weight of your body to push your knee towards the bench.

4.   **Relax**
     Exhaling:

     • Hold the knee in a comfortable position, either with your hand or by itself.

     • Let it find its "new normal".

     • Breathe and relax in that position.

Sitting Forward Bend (hips, glutes, and hamstrings)

After moving your knee toward the bench, the next step is to bend forward. This movement stretches the hips, adding pressure to the knee at the same time.

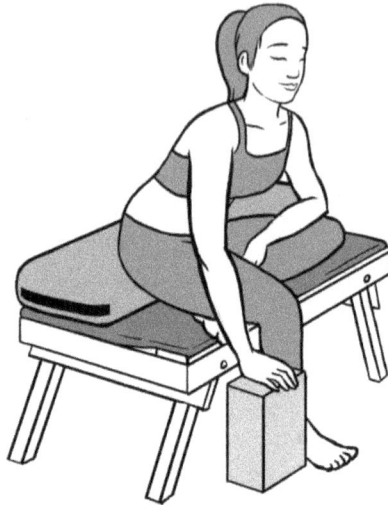

When both feet are on the floor, that means bending forward with your knees together, or out ahead of you in line with your hips.

In Half Tibetan and Half Butterfly positions, it means bending forward with the other knee (the one with the foot on the floor) straight ahead.

In those positions, you're mostly stretching the hips, the glutes (backside), and hamstrings.

Quarter Lotus pose is the exception. It's okay to keep the other knee straight ahead if you can do it comfortably, but for most of us that leg will need to be angled to the side. In that position, the foot rests on the soft inner thigh instead of directly on the thigh bone, which most of us find a lot more comfortable for the upper foot.

Ideally, you have Yoga Blocks positioned at each side of the bench. As you bend forward, now is the time to grab them and put them on the floor ahead of you.

You can also control your degree of movement by placing your hands or even your elbows on your knees.

As always, you can simply breathe and relax in this position, or go through the Movement Sequence for an increased stretch.

Sitting Angled Bend (hip, groin, and thigh rotation)

In this asana, you bend forward at an angle.

When both feet are on the floor, move them so the knees are angled outward, wide enough that your shoulders fit between them. You will now be stretching the groin and encouraging a thigh rotation as you bend forward.

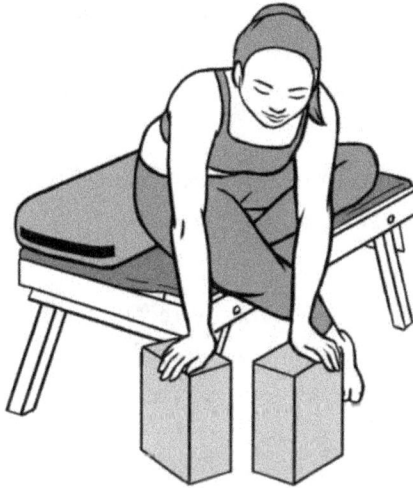

You can also do it with a single Yoga Block, as shown on the next page.

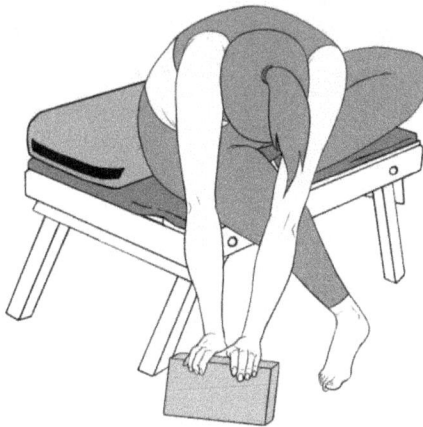

In most other positions, one foot is "on top" and the other is "down". For this step, bend towards the foot that is on top—or more exactly, over the thigh that is next to it.

The full Tibetan Pose is the one position where there is no "top" foot. Instead, one foot is in front of the other. For that pose, consider your front foot as the one on top. (That's the one you can move most easily, and if you place it anywhere else, it will be on top.)

With this bend, you are isolating the hip you're stretching away from, stretching the groin a bit. To encourage a *rotation* of the thigh you're stretching away from, put your hand on it, push down, and rotate it outward.

This is another great move I learned from David Keil in another of his YouTube videos, Preparation for Lotus.

> Note:
> The "Double Pigeon" asana he recommends is great, but it requires a lot of flexibility. One alternative is to sit on a bolster and put one foot up on a Yoga Block, as he recommends. But sitting on the bench, in Half Tibetan position, you get the very same stretch for each leg, one at a time—*without* the need for the substantial amount of flexibility that is needed just to get into position.
>
> He also recommends holding each pose for 5 to 15 breaths. That's a decent range. I find 7 or 8 to be really effective, and often stop after 5. But I breathe fairly slowly. By all means, do whatever works best for you!

Finishing Sequence

After sitting for a while, the legs and back get tight. This short sequence takes less than a minute, but it works like magic to restore fluidity to your body. If you have done the sitting flexibility exercises and have sat in meditation for a while, you are probably ready for these.

As your practice grows, you will add more asanas and exercises, and you will sit longer in meditation, experiencing energy flows and "communing". But at the end of the practice, after your final "Namaste", this is the way to bring flexibility back to a stiffened body.

Basic Movements

1. **Standing forward bend**

   - To make it extra effective, use the Dynamic Subtle Energy Sequence described earlier. But you can also just "hang out" for a while. That's the first step in the movement sequence, in any case.

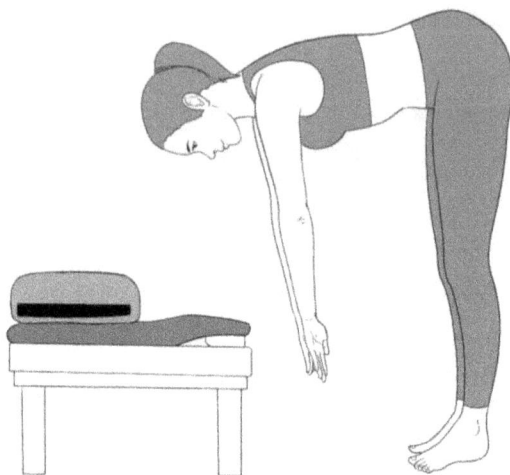

2. **Upward Arch (head up)**

   I like to inhale during this movement:

   - From the forward bend, move to an arms-overhead position.

     ▪ If your back allows it, interlace your fingers and, with your arms straight, arch your back and move directly upward. This mini-deadlift helps to strengthen the back muscles, so it's my favorite move.

       Important:
       Arch your lower back as you do this move. When it is arched, the strain is on your hamstrings and glutes, rather than your back. When your back is bent, the strain is on your back muscles.

       Learn more: Kinesiology of Exercise, by Dr. Michael Yessis, pp. 31-37.

     ▪ For a safer movement, bring your arms out to the sides and up, in a reverse Swan Dive. You can still keep your back straight for a mini-deadlift that has less weight.

     ▪ For the ultimate in safety, curl up one vertebrae at a time, keeping your hands close to your body.

   - At the top, arch your back and look up at the ceiling.

     ▪ A study of biomechanics tells me that position produces the 30-degree arch that the spine is capable of.

     ▪ Of course, it is possible to bend back farther—but the only way to do it is to push your hips forward, to counterbalance the movement.

     ▪ What's important to understand about that move is that you are *not* bending

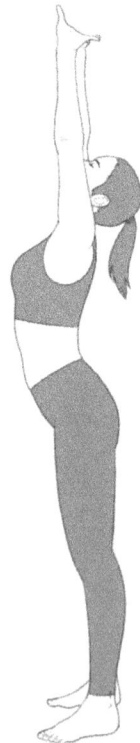

your spine any more than you were before. All you have done really, is to increase the pressure on your lower back.

- If you're a gymnast, you may have good reasons for making that move. But if you're just trying to arch your spine to stretch your back, there is no point.

- So if you feel your hips moving forward as you arch your back, you're arching too far!

- *Note:*
  Observation tells me women can bend backward more easily, maybe to where they're looking at the back corner of the ceiling, where it meets the wall.

  That extra flexibility could be due to skeletal structure, or the lack of flexibility in the male anatomy could be due to extra musculature in the torso—the kind you need to carry a bear back to the den. But for whatever reason, women seem to bend backward farther and more easily. The lesson for men is: Don't try to keep up with the women on this stretch! So for a standing arch, I recommend keeping your hips in place.

3. **Buddha Arch (head down)**
   I like to exhale during this one:

   - With fingers still interlaced overhead, drop your head and look at your toes.

   - This move transfers the stretch from the back to the *trapezius*—a triangular muscle that runs from between your shoulder blades up and out to your shoulders, alongside your neck.

4. **Arm Circles**
   I'll inhale again for this one:

   - Keeping the arms straight, pull them down and out to the sides at shoulder level.

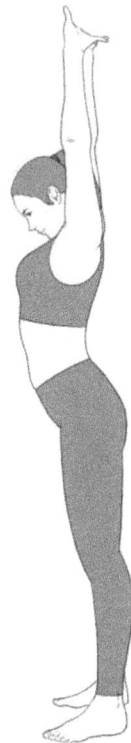

- Make fists and rotate your arms in small circles.

- I like to rotate up and back, down and forward.

- You can rotate the other way, too, if you want. (If you do, do that first.) But for most of us, our shoulders already slump too much. "Up and back" produces the stretch we really need.

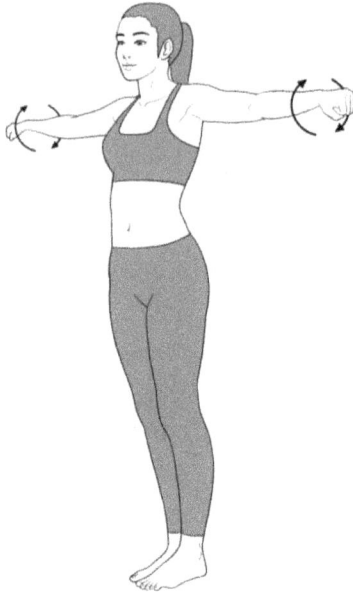

5. **Arms Back**

   When I've finished inhaling, I'll exhale for this movement. Then I'll stay in it for another inhalation.

   - Interlace fingers behind your back.

   - Push them away from you and lift them upward as far as you can comfortably, without leaning forward.

   - This move stretches the front of the shoulders and the chest, while you arch your back—all important for good posture.

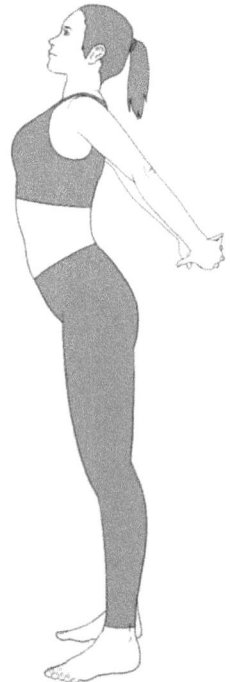

Additional Movements

Do these additional steps for shoulder flexibility, if you feel inclined:

6. **Behind the back elbow grab**
    - Fold your arms behind you at your lower back.
    - Grasp elbows if you can, or grasp forearms.
    - Breathe and give a slight pull.
    - For a better stretch, grasp one wrist or forearm at a time, pulling it across your body and lifting it upward.

7. **Up and down hands behind back**
    - One arm goes over your head and down behind it.
    - The other comes up from your lower back.
    - The goal is to join hands at the shoulder blades.
    - Get as close as you can, breathe, and inch a bit further.

8. **Doorway Sequence**
    I learned from my chiropractor, Helen Shaw. Along with the Supported Back Bend, these are great for expanding the chest and stretching out the front of the shoulders.

    a) **One arm lunge**.
    - One arm high on the doorframe, above your head.
    - Lunge forward to stretch the shoulder.
    - Bend your rear knee to drop lower, increasing the stretch.

    b) **Arms overhead**.
    - Both arms straight up in front of the doorframe, so they extend beyond it.
    - Lean forward, so your arms stretch out back behind your head.

    c) **Elbows out.**

- Arms at shoulder height, one elbow on each side of the doorframe.
- Forearms can be straight up, or anywhere they are comfortable.
- Lean forward, stretching your chest and shoulders.

Joint Rotation Warmup

Joint rotations are a great way to get the body warmed up, and ready to sit. In Shivananda Yoga, they're called "Subtle Yoga" because, in addition to bringing nutrients to the joints, these movements clear the pathways for subtle energy flows through the body.

These take only a minute or so. I like to do them top-down, in the sequence shown here but you can do them in any sequence that appeals to you. For example, you can do them from the bottom up. Or you can do them alternating upper and lower, starting at the middle and working out, or starting at the head and toes and then moving towards the center.

For an even better warmup, I recommend the *Sitting Warmups* described in the next chapter. Those movements include these joint rotations, but with an extra "subtle energy" dimension. (That sequence has replaced this one, in my personal practice. But I'm leaving this section in as a quick-reference outline for those who can use it.)

1. Light neck rotations
2. Head side to side
3. Head twist
4. Shoulder squeezes: Up, Down, Shoulder Blades together
5. Shoulder rotations
6. Side bends
7. Chest side to side
8. Torso rotations
    - Chest and shoulders circle around as though scraping the inside of a barrel.
9. Torso twist
    - One hand pushing on opposite knee.
    - Other hand behind you, gently pulling on the seat cushion.
10. Upper thigh rotations in hip socket

11. Pump the Brake
    - While sitting on the floor, bend and straighten one leg at a time, as though driving a car, when you lift your leg off the gas pedal and move it to the brake.
12. Ankle bend and straighten
13. Ankle rotations
14. Bend and straighten toes, with ankles bent
15. Hands alternately straighten and make fists
16. Fingers spread and pressed together in prayer position
17. Backs of wrists pressed together, elbows out
18. Wrist twists, Aikido style
    a. Fingers up, palm to outside, opposite thumb below pinky, fingers grasp base of thumb.
    b. Palm facing away, opposite fingers grasp edge of hand.

Sitting Warmups

You don't have to warm up, of course. You can sit for meditation and listen to your inner guidance for a sense of what to do—or not do—in your current session. But warming up is a good way to get the energy moving—and energy is the foundation of great meditations—so I recommend it.

These movements seem simple, but they help the subtle energies move through the joints, rather than getting stuck there. They also lubricate the joints, so they work better. And, as you'll see, at times you will be squeezing muscles in ways that will improve strength *around* the joints, as well.

> *Note:*
> Some of these actions may cause muscles to cramp. If they do, see the section on Handling Cramps in the Personal Practice chapter.

Muscle-Squeeze Isotonics

An *isotonic* exercise is one where you simply squeeze the muscles in some area of the body—all of the muscles in that area, as hard as you can. You're not working against any resistance, you are simply activating your muscles.

These exercises activate the muscles and get the blood flowing, the same way cats do when they stretch after sleeping. In fact, these exercises are a great way to wake up in the morning, before you even get out of bed!

Once you get up, you may be inspired to continue squeezing practices, adding in a few cat-like stretches. But most of the benefit comes from the squeezing action itself. You'll learn all about those benefits in a later chapter. For now, just follow along to wake up your body and get your practice started.

Squeezing and the Breath

When squeezing a muscle, I use the breath mostly as a *timing* device. I generally squeeze while exhaling, but it is perfectly fine to squeeze while inhaling, instead. It is even possible to squeeze during the pause *between* breaths.

Which variation I use depends on the time needed for the movements.

For example, it takes no time at all to transition from a head-back position to a head-forward position. So I begin inhaling as I move my head back, and begin squeezing as soon as my head comes to rest. Then I'll relax and begin exhaling as I move my head forward, and squeeze until I finish exhaling. I'll use the same breath timing for Cat/Cow poses.

The Torso Twist, on the other hand, takes more time. For that, I'll exhale and squeeze as I twist in one direction, then relax and inhale as I come back to center, and finally exhale and squeeze as I twist to the other side.

Neck Squeeze

The neck muscles need strength to hold your head up, centered over your spine. If the neck muscles are weak, your head drops forward into the "chicken neck" position that slumps your shoulders and bends your spine.

Although it isn't the largest muscle used to maintain an erect posture, it is still an important one. And it is easy to exercise.

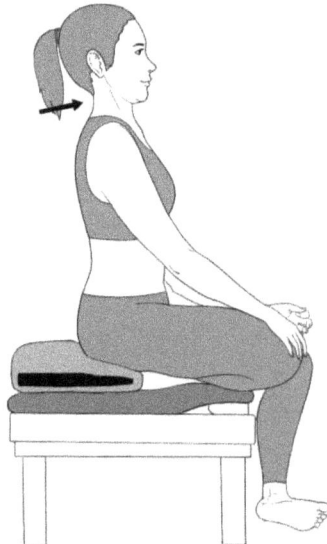

This is something of a strengthening exercise, of course, but it's easy to do—and it's a great way to warm up neck muscles for the activities ahead.

1.   Start by taking a deep breath.

2.   As you exhale, squeeze every muscle in your neck as hard as you can.

3.   When you're done exhaling, release the tension.

That's all there is to it! This form of exercise is also known as "dynamic tension"—especially when a body part is moving, as opposed to standing still. The concept was popularized by Charles Atlas in the early 1900's, and was also introduced to the West as part of Yoga training by Yogananda. (Which came first, I would love to know!)

Personally, I like the name *Dynamic Tension*. But "tension" is a dirty word these days, so for now we will call this kind of exercise *isotonic* (*iso*, "same", as in "same position" and *tonic*, as "tones and invigorates"). Alternatively, we'll call them "*muscle squeeze*" exercises.

Upper Back Squeeze

Just like the Neck Isotonic:

1.   Take a deep breath.

2.   As you exhale, squeeze your upper back as hard as you can.

3.   When you're done exhaling, release the tension.

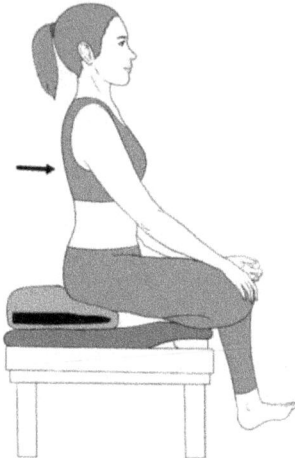

Lower Back Squeeze

Just like the upper back squeeze, only focusing on the lower back. Squeeze the muscles of your lower back and core as you exhale. Give it everything you have.

Abdominal Squeeze

Exhale, pulling your belly in and up. Squeeze as hard as you can until you need to breathe, then release the tension.

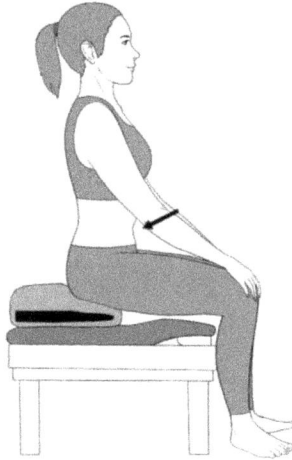

Other Squeezes

Depending on time and how I feel, I'll squeeze other muscles as well:

- Chest, Arms, Abdomen
- Forearms
- Pelvis, Thighs
- Calves

I'll have a lot more to say about such exercises in a later volume in this series. For now, just use your imagination. Create!

Neck

Forward and Back

- Bend your head forward, tucking the chin into your clavicle rather than pushing it down your chest.
- At the end of your range of motion, squeeze the muscles you are using, pushing in as hard as you can.
- Pull your head back so you're looking up at the ceiling.
- At the end, squeeze the neck muscles, pulling back as much as you can..

Note:
For this kind of movement, I like to inhale as I come out of a position, exhale as I'm going into the next position, and squeeze as I finish exhaling.

Side to Side

- Push your ear down to your shoulder. Pull your shoulder down at the same time, so it's not rising up to meet your ear.
- At the end of your range of motion, squeeze the muscles you are using, pushing down as hard as you can.
- Repeat to the other side.

Twist

- Turn your head to the side.
- At the end of your range of motion, squeeze the muscles you are using, twisting as hard as you can.
- Repeat to the other side.

Chiropractic Lift

- o Lift your chin up and to the side.
- o At the end of your range of motion, squeeze the muscles you are using, lifting as hard as you can.
- o Repeat to the other side.

Rotations

- o Bend your head forward. Rotate it to the side, back, and around to the front.
- o Go back the other way.
- o Repeat a couple of times.

Shoulders

Shoulders to Ears

- o Pull both shoulders upward, so they touch your head behind your ears.
- o At the end of your range of motion, squeeze the muscles you are using, pulling your shoulders up as hard as you can.

Shoulder Blades Together

- o Pull your shoulder blades down and back, as though trying to make them touch each other.
- o At the end of your range of motion, squeeze the muscles you are using, pulling your shoulder blades together as hard as you can.

Rotations

- o Rotate your shoulders up and back, then down and to the front.

- ○ That motion stretches and loosens the tendons at the front of the shoulder.

- ○ There is no need to go the other way. Our shoulders have plenty of flexibility in the opposite direction. (We slump our shoulders too much in our daily life!)

Fingers and Wrists

I got the first finger and wrist movements from Pat Laster's great video, Easy Yoga (for Seniors). You can ignore the "for seniors" part. Trust me. It's great. Well-paced, meditative, and instructional. A great introduction to Yoga. (As mentioned in the Resources, you can find it on YouTube, and you can get old VHS copies at Amazon.)

The Aikido stretches are particularly good, too. I've never seen them anywhere else, so I'm including them here. (Full disclosure: I never studied Aikido. But I read a book and liked the principles. The wrist stretches are one aspect of the practice that stuck with me.)

Finger Pad Press & Fist Squeeze

- ○ Spread fingers wide. Press the pads of the fingers together.

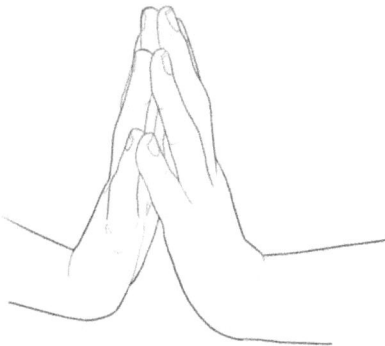

- ○ Start at chin height. Increase the pressure by bringing your hands down, and elbows out to the side.

- ○ No additional squeezing is needed for this stretch.

o   After pressing the fingers together, make fists with palms up.

o   Squeeze them as hard as you can.

o   Repeat the sequence: Fingertip Press followed by Fist Squeeze

Open Fingers

o   After your last fist squeeze, open the fingers as wide as you can, and pull them back as far as you can.

o   At the end of your range of motion, squeeze the muscles you are using, straightening your fingers and pulling them back as hard as you can.

Aikido Bend (forward and back)

o   Use one hand to gently push on the back of your wrist, bending it towards your forearm.

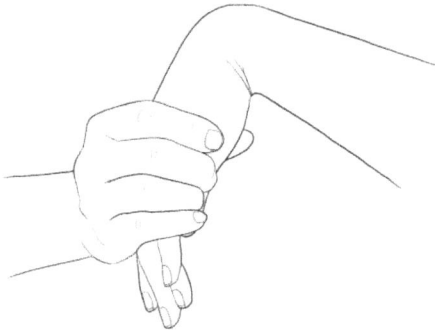

o   There is no muscle squeezing during this movement. The other hand provides more than enough pressure.

o   You can also use one hand to push the palm of the other, pushing the back of the hand towards the forearm.

Aikido Wrist Twists

○   Put one hand up in front of your chest, rotating it so the palm is facing outward towards your shoulder. Put the thumb of the other hand at the base of the small fingers, then curl your fingers around the base of the thumb and apply pressure to twist the wrist.

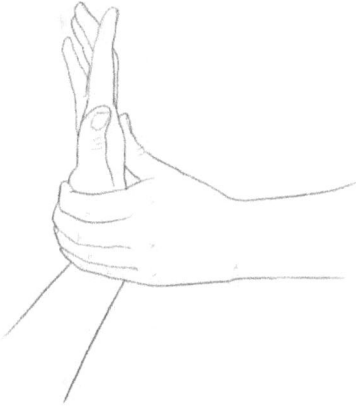

○   Face the palm outward with thumb down. Curl the fingers of your other hand over the top, around the edge of the hand. Put your thumb at the base of the large fingers and apply pressure to twist the wrist in the opposite direction.

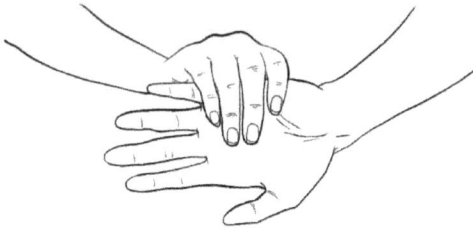

○   There is no muscle squeezing during these movements. The other hand provides more than enough pressure.

Rotations

○   Make fists and rotate your wrists, first in one direction, then the other.

Spine

Seated Cat/Cow

The good old "Cat/Cow" position, or as Pat Laster likes to called it, "Stretching Cat/Angry Cat", done in a seated position:

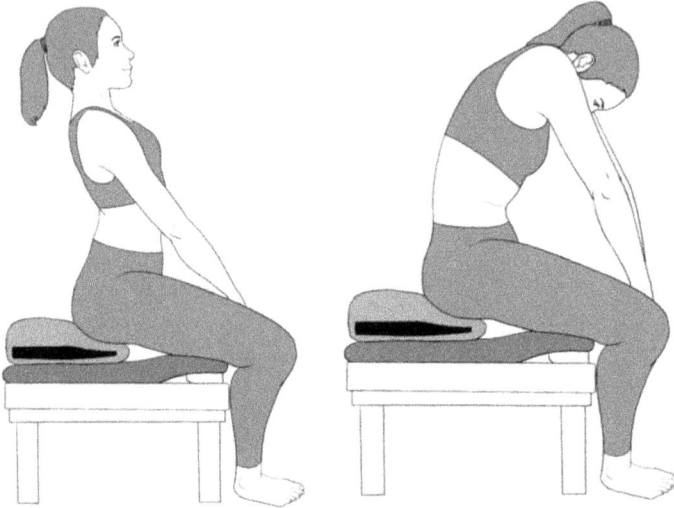

- o   As you come forward, round your shoulders, as well as your back.

- o   As you come back, pull back your shoulders, squeezing the shoulder blades together.

Side Bend

- o   Push your shoulder down towards your hip.

- o   At the end of your range of motion, squeeze the muscles you are using, pushing your shoulder down as hard as you can.

- o   Repeat on the other side.

Side-to-Side Chest

- ○ Keeping shoulders level, push chest and shoulders to one side.
- ○ At the end of your range of motion, squeeze the muscles you are using, pushing to the side as hard as you can.
- ○ Repeat on the other side.

Chest Circles

- ○ Keeping your hips and shoulders as still as possible, rotate your chest and diaphragm in circles, as though you were scraping the inside of the barrel.
- ○ Repeat in the opposite direction.

Torso Twist

- ○ Put one hand on the opposite knee, the other on the seat cushion behind you. Twist your torso.
- ○ At the end of your range of motion, squeeze the muscles you are using, twisting your shoulders as hard as you can.
- ○ Repeat on the other side.

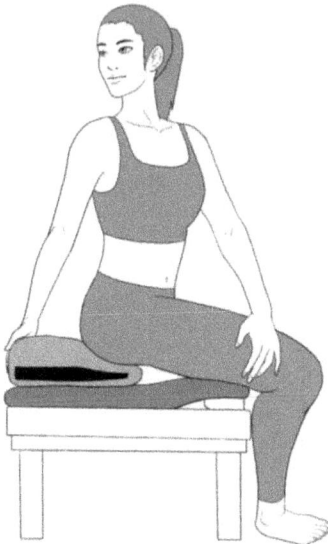

Spine Wave

- This movement is easier to demonstrate than it is to describe!

- Start by bending your head and chest forward as your lower back moves backward.

- Push your diaphragm forward as your head comes down more deeply to your chest.

- Push your chest forward as your head starts lifting.

- As your head reaches the end of its upward lift, the lower back moves backward, and the sequence starts again.

- Do it a few times. In time, you'll get a nice wave-movement going.

    Note:
    I developed this practice after using my chiropractor's "Wave Machine". It's a bench you lie on while a roller moves up and down your spine, pushing first one part up, then the next. (It's a great machine that is extremely effective! This exercise lets us simulate the motion to some degree, at least.)

Hip Joints

Leg Circles

- With the toes of your foot on the ground and your heel in the air, rotate your thigh and knee in circles. Imagine there is a clock in front of the knee. Trace the face of the clock with your knee, following the path of the minute hand.

- Rotate first in one direction, then the other

- Repeat with the other leg.

Knees

Brake Pedals

○ Slide feet back and forth on the floor, gently moving the knees as though pressing on a brake pedal.

○ You can also lean back slightly and keep your feet in the air, but there will be more strengthening exercises of that kind later on, so there is no real need to do it now.

○ There is no squeezing in this movement. It's a simple joint movement.

Ankles & Toes

Ankle Lift and Extend

○ Lift your ankles, bending them back towards your shins.

○ At the end of your range of motion, squeeze the muscles you are using, pulling your feet back as hard as you can.

○ Straighten your ankles to point your toes.

○ At the end of your range of motion, squeeze the muscles you are using, pushing your feet forward as hard as you can.

○ Repeat a couple of times.

Toe Lift and Curl

○ With ankles straight, pull your toes back toward your shins.

○ At the end of your range of motion, squeeze the muscles you are using, pulling your toes back as hard as you can.

○ Curl your toes as though using them to pick up a pencil.

- o   At the end of your range of motion, squeeze the muscles you are using, curling your toes as hard as you can.

- o   Repeat a couple of times.

Note:
Curling the toes helps to strengthen the arch, as well

Ankle Rotations

- o   Rotate your ankles with heels on the floor.

- o   For extra abdominal work, hold your feet in the air.

- o   Repeat in the opposite direction.

Eyes, Gums, Face

This is an optional "super subtle" sequence of movements that help to keep you healthy. They improve eyesight, help to keep teeth and gums strong, and keep you looking young.

Eyes

It can help to do these sequences by following the tip of your thumb. Hold it at arm's length in front of you, at the level of your eyes. Then move it in the indicated direction, following the movement with your eyes.

Note:
I learned that technique from visiting teacher Radheshyam Mishra (RSM) who created the DVD, 24 Minutes Yoga for 24 Hours of Energy. He reported that by doing it twice a day, he was able to discard his glasses. Doing them once a day should help you avoid the expense of stronger prescriptions, at the very least.

You can also do the exercises as isometrics, simply pushing your eyes in the indicated direction as hard as you can.

○ **Near Focus**

- With eyes focused normally, about three feet in front of you, pull them in until you are focused on the tip of your nose.

- At the end of your range of motion, squeeze the muscles you are using, focusing your eyes as hard as you can.

- Return your eyes to a normal focus, then repeat the sequence, this time focusing on the point between your eyebrows.

- Return your eyes to a normal focus, and repeat once again, this time focusing at the point between your eyes, at the bridge of the nose.

○ **Far Focus**

- With eyes focused normally, about three feet in front of you, push them outward until you are focusing on a far away mountain.

- At the end of your range of motion, squeeze the muscles you are using, focusing your eyes as hard as you can.

○ **General Strengthening**

- For each of the 8 directions (up/down, left/right, and diagonals), push both eyes in that direction.

- At the end of your range of motion, squeeze the muscles you are using, pushing your eyes in that direction as hard as you can.

Tip:
You can do similar eye-isometrics while doing standard Yoga asanas—eyes up when you arch back, eyes down when you bend forward, and eyes to the side when you twist.

Gums

○   It is a truism among dental health professionals that bone loss in the area of the gums is permanent—that it never grows back. But I suspect that their belief is not quite accurate.

○   You see, bone grows when a) The required nutrients are present (so a good diet is essential) and b) *When muscular stress is applied to the bone.*

○   Without muscular stress, the bone does not grow, or even maintain its strength. It just grows weaker, over time. (More women need weight training than know about it, for that very reason.)

○   Once you have begun to isolate small muscles in the body and begin to squeeze them, it becomes possible to identify the very small muscles that attach your gums to the bones underneath them.

○   If you squeeze those muscles, and your nutrition is good, you should be able to grow new bone in those areas. (It will take tests to be sure, but it's worth a try! I've been doing it, but don't have good before/after x-rays I can use to gauge progress. At the very least, it does no harm. At best, it can make a big difference. We know that bone in the gums *does* grow—that's how braces work! Adding a bit of muscle tension can only help.)

Face

This exercise comes from Fumiko Takatsu's book, The Ultimate Guide to the Face Yoga Method. (This one is on the cover of the book.)

○   Lift your eyebrows as high as you can.

○   At the same time, drop your jaw and mouth an "O".

○   At the end of your range of motion, squeeze the muscles you are using, raising your eyebrows as far as you can, and making the strongest   "O"   you   can

Bench Warmups

These two warmups help get you ready for sitting positions.

Weaker Leg Acclimation

Some of us have two weak legs. Some have two strong legs. But almost all of us have one leg that is stronger than the other!

When I sit for an initial meditation, and do the sitting warmups, I almost always sit with my stronger leg up on the bench. It's the more comfortable way to sit!

But after doing that, the weaker leg needs a chance to catch up. For me, that is the right leg.

To ease into it, I'll start by sitting with that foot up on the bench, with the other knee raised.

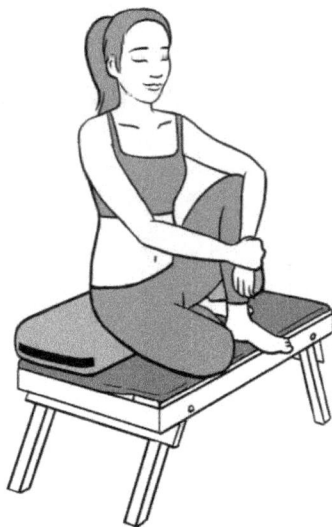

In that position, much of your body weight is on the hip, which minimizes pressure on the knee.

Then I will put the upper knee down, with the thigh over towards in the knee, in a position that puts the least pressure on the weaker knee when the foot is on the ground:

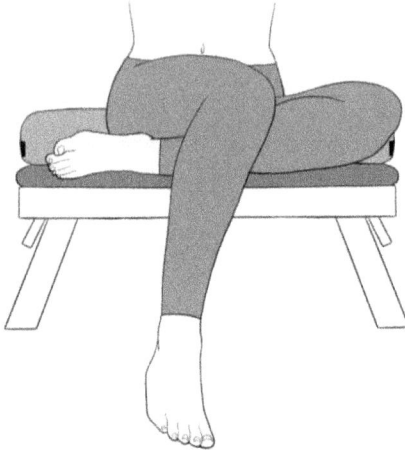

Then comes the intermediate position, with the thigh over the heel:

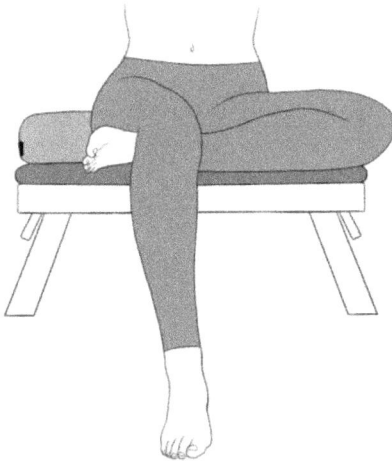

The hips are closer to level now, which increases pressure on the knee.

If things feel good, I'll move to the wide-spread position, with the thigh cradled in the arch of the foot, as shown on the next page:

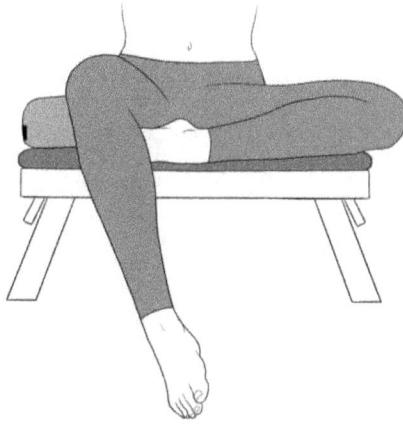

The hips are now totally level, and the pelvis has begun to tilt. The back is feeling more comfortable, as a result, but the weaker knee is also feeling more pressure.

In that position, I'll generally start with my foot out, in the easier, "on edge" position:

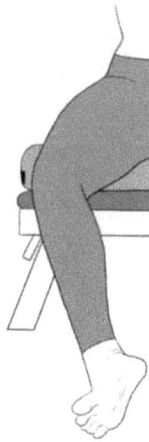

Pulling the foot straight back from that position puts the foot flat on the floor and angled outwards, but since the foot is still out to side the pelvic tilt and knee pressure remain constant.

From there, I'll gradually pull the foot inward to one of the stronger positions, as shown on the next page:

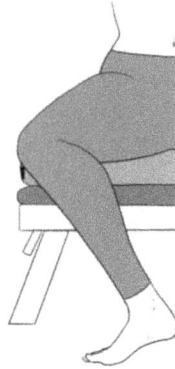

As the foot comes into the centerline and beyond (with heel raised), the tilt of the pelvis increases and posture becomes more upright.

In my case, the stronger knee doesn't feel any pressure in that position, because it is fully supported by the bench and because the cartilage is basically intact. But in my weaker leg, where some of the cartilage was surgically removed, pressure is felt in each position.

The good news is that the lack of cartilage forced me to discover the sitting-position variations, and made it easy to discern their effects. (The better news is that I have at last found a way to *regrow* that cartilage, prompted by the first 4 minutes of Dr. John Berman's YouTube video, How to Regenerate Joints.)

Bench Vajrasana

In standard Yoga, *vajrasana* is the position where you kneel on the floor, rotate your ankles outward, and then sit on the tops of your feet, with your backside nestled between your heels. It's a great pose, if you have the flexibility to do it.

What *makes* it such a great pose is the way it lets you find the perfectly balanced, perfectly upright position for your back. Nothing is quite as comfortable for your back—if your legs can stand it.

The short (9 inch) bench used for Japanese *zazen* (Zen meditation) can make it easier. You can sit on it, or move it forward so it is under your thighs. Or you can sit on a cushion, to make it easier.

But for some of us, that still isn't enough!

To get more height, we can put a Yoga Block on top of the cushion we're sitting on, or we can simply kneel in front of the bench and sit back against the edge.

That "tall vajrasana" position doesn't put any pressure to speak of on the knees. So it's a comfortable way to meditate after the weaker-leg acclimation process.

There are many good times to use it, too:

○ It's good after the Standing Warmups (coming next), to transition back to the bench.

○ It's a good way to start the Bench Asanas (coming later), since it really is a bench-specific asana—one you cannot easily do any other way.

○ It's good anytime you want to sit with your back fully relaxed while giving your legs a break.

Later, you'll see the Leaning Vajrasana that helps progress towards this important pose. But when sitting normally (without leaning forward) you can use this progression to measure your progress (approximately):

1. Edge of bench with a base cushion and another small cushion—14 inches

2. Edge of bench with base cushion—12 inches

3. Cushion on your calves with a Yoga Block on top—10 inches

4. Japanese Zazen Bench under your thighs—9 inches

5. Japanese Zazen Bench, sitting—8 inches

6. Large rectangular bolster (the seat cushion) on your calves —7 inches

7. Small rectangular bolster (the support cushion) on your calves—6 inches

Standing Warmups

There are many possible ways to warm up. This is one sequence I happen to like. We start with some standing positions, and then move to sitting rotations.

Standing Cat/ Cow

This is a great way to start. It stretches the hamstrings and back, and begins to get the blood flowing.

1. Start by doing a forward fold with hands on the bench, in *Standing Table* pose.

2. Put block on the bench if you need more height, or put the block on the floor if you can go lower while keeping your back flat.

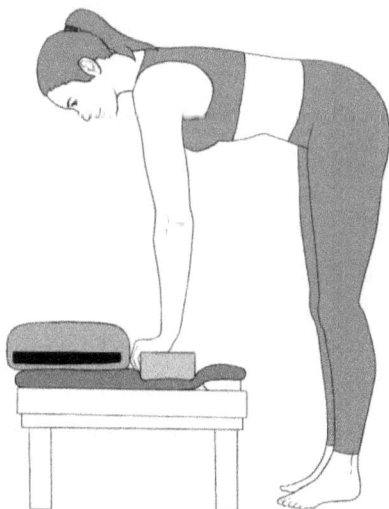

3. Arch your back as you inhale, lifting your head and dropping your stomach.

4. At the end of your range of motion, squeeze the muscles you are using, arching your back as hard as you can.

5. Round your back as you exhale, dropping your head, pulling in your stomach, and raising your shoulder blades towards the ceiling.

6. At the end of your range of motion, squeeze the muscles you are using, pushing your back upward as hard as you can.

High Squats

Light squats, with your knees going halfway to the bench, or a little more. The idea is mostly to move the joint, rather than to exercise the legs. (This is a warmup!)

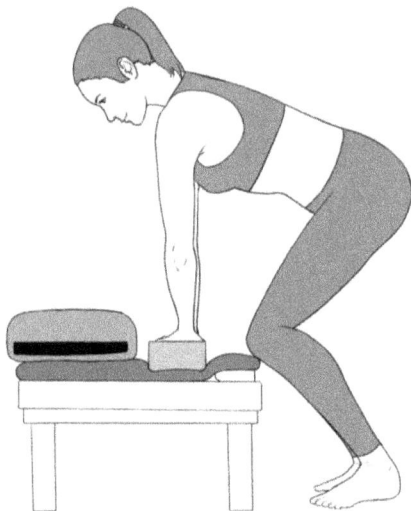

For a bit more exercise you can stand upright, but the general idea is to simply move the knees without any real pressure on them.

Twenty or 30 of them take less than a minute, with no real strain. (You bend deeper to sit in a chair.) It's a great way to get the blood flowing, especially in the hip, knee, and ankle joints.

To minimize strain, use the bench or block for support. Or stand up straight for a bit more of a workout.

Knee (and ankle) Rotations

1. Feet together, hands on the bench, or a block, or the knees. You can get more exercise by putting your hands on your knees, but I find that I get a much better range of motion with my hands on a block, on the bench, as in the High Squat above.

2. Go into a mild squat.

3. Keep your head level as you rotate knees around to the side, straightening your legs as they come under you.

4. As you go deeper, roll onto the edges of your feet as your knees go around, extending the rotation to your ankles.

Pyramid Pose

A great stretch that works the hamstrings, one at a time. Use the bench for balance.

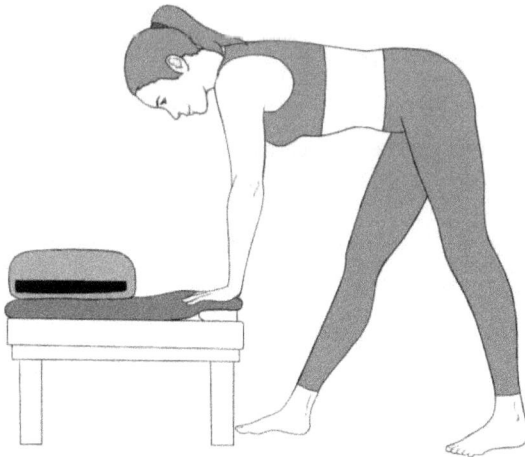

Block-Standing Calf Stretch

When calves are tight, hamstring stretches become a lot more difficult. So before stretching the hamstrings, it helps to loosen the calves. (I wasn't aware of just *how much* difference it made, until recently. Once I saw the difference, this stretch and the next one became a regular part of the series.)

1. Put a Yoga Block on the floor in front of the bench, in its lowest orientation.

2. Lean forward and put your hands on the bench for balance. (For more height, put a Yoga Block on the bench.)

3. Stand on the edge of the Yoga Block with both feet.

   - The ball of each foot is on the block. The arch and the heel are hanging off.

   - I have large feet, and they still fit. And somewhat surprisingly, the block doesn't tip over! (But it's helpful to have it on a soft surface, in any case.)

4. Let one heel drop down.

   - To increase the stretch, wrap you other leg around the back of your ankle.

   - At your farthest stretch, use muscular effort to push down as hard as you can.

5. Repeat with the other leg.

6. Drop both heels down and bounce a bit.

   - Don't bounce too hard, but do give your calves a little bouncing action.

7. For an optional *plyometric* (explosion) exercise, when you get to the bottom of a bounce immediately lift upward, using your calves to raise yourself as high as you can. Then bounce and explode upward again, repeating a few times.

   - The calves are an important of running speed and jump height.

   - They were designed for this kind of fast, instantaneous movement. This exercise gives it to them.

Balancing Hamstring Stretch

This movement is a balance pose that warms up the standing leg at the same time that it stretches the hamstring of the active leg, preparing it for the more active stretches to come.

1. Stand facing the bench.
2. Put the heel of one foot on the bench—leg straight, toes up.
3. Lean forward over that leg to stretch the hamstrings.
4. As you exhale, *squeeze* the muscles in your support leg. That action strengthens the small muscles that help you keep your balance.

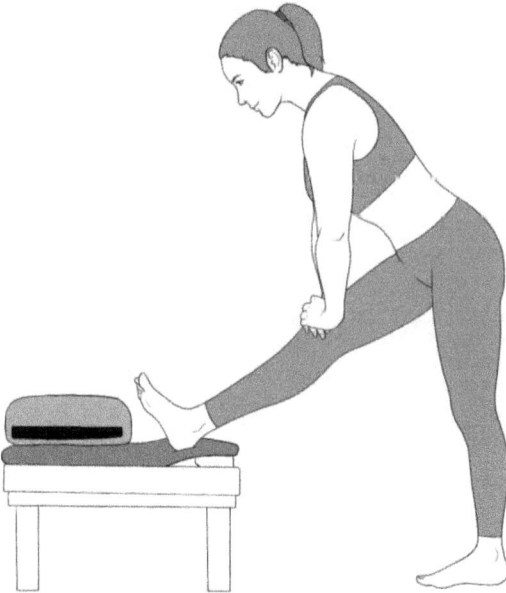

Down Dog / Up Dog

Just like the floor version, but using the bench. Good for the hamstrings and calves.

Here is Down Dog:

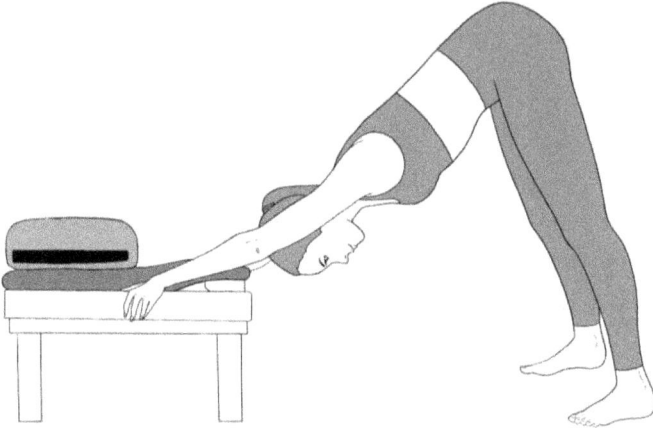

And here is Up Dog:

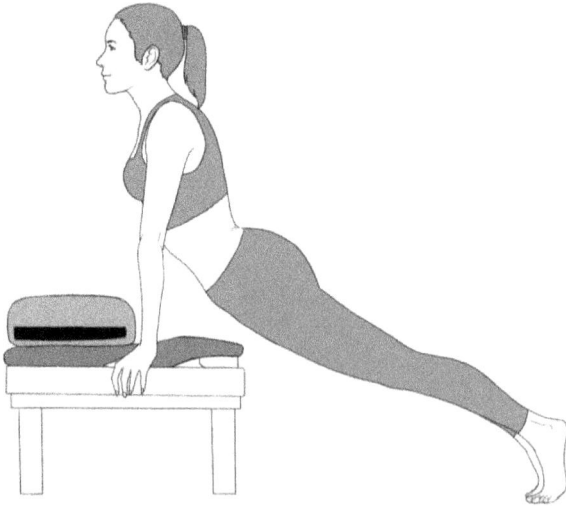

Squat

1. Face the bench. Use it for support and for balance.
2. Keep heels on the floor. Go as low as you can. Hold as long as you can, comfortably.
3. Lean towards the bench for support coming up.
4. Warms up the leg muscles and flexes the knee joints.

   Note:

   In a normal yoga practice, you press the elbows against the insides of the knees to push them outward. With the bench, you can get the same effect more easily by putting your hands at the sides of the bench with your elbows against your knees. You still press outward, but you have the bench for balance.

Straddle Split

With the bench and optional Yoga Block(s) for support, this otherwise difficult pose becomes quite easy. It's a great stretch for the groin that makes sitting positions easier, and you can get to your perfect "edge" position (not too little, and not too much).

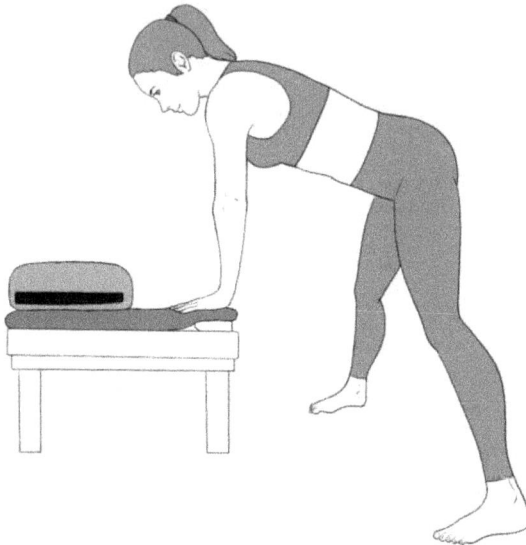

Until you're pretty flexible, even a Yoga Block is pretty far out of reach, when it's on the floor. The Yoga Bench gives you a great way to get the support you need to keep from over-stressing the groin as you stretch, because it gives you perfect control over the degree of pressure in the stretch.

1. Prepare by putting a Yoga Block or two on the bench, if needed.

2. Lean forward onto the bench (with optional blocks), and walk your feet out to the sides, heel-toe fashion.

3. Lean forward to take more weight on your hands.

4. Work the Yoga Block(s) to higher positions to move your body back over your legs, adding more weight to the stretch.

5. You can increase the stretch by raising your torso to an upright position, for as long as you can hold it there comfortably.

6. You can also increase the stretch by taking your torso lower, with this progression:

    - Elbows down to the bench

    - Arms folded on the bench, head resting on arms

    - Hands to the floor (put a Yoga Block on the floor, if needed)

    - Head to the bench (or to your folded arms on the bench)

Alternating Lunge

This is a great warmup for the Side-to-Side Squat that's coming next. In fact, when called upon to perform martial arts demonstrations, many of the advanced students I trained with used this movement and the upcoming straddle squats to warm up.

The movements are incredibly effective for warming up the groin and hamstrings, but can be difficult to do without a support. The bench makes them much easier.

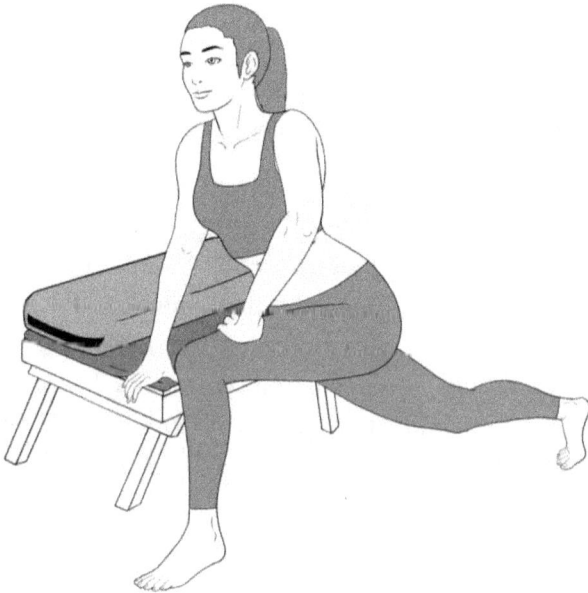

To perform the Alternating Lunge:

1. From a standing position, face the bunch and lunge to the left.

2. Or, from a straddle:

   - With your hands on the bench, pull your left foot in until the foot is under the knee.

   - The center of the knee should be directly over the ankle bone. Not ahead of it or behind it, and not to either side.

   - Twist your body to face your foot, lifting the right heel in the process so you come up onto the ball of the foot.

3. Put your right palm on the bench for support.

    - For maximum comfort in the fingers and wrist, curl your fingers over the edge of the bench.

    - Put a Yoga block on the bench for more height.

    - Or put it on the floor to go lower.

4. Left hand or elbow is on your knee.

5. Adjust your rear leg to go lower or higher, until the top of thigh is parallel to the floor.

6. Walk your hands to the other side of the bench and lunge to the right.

When you're done with the lunge, your feet are the perfect distance apart for the Side-to-Side Squat, which comes next.

> *Note:*
>
> This warm up exercise and the next are done with a mild *bounce*. That's a different kind of movement, for people used to static stretching (and who buy into the theory). But ligaments that have been elongated can still be stiff! If they are, they are still prone to injury. A mild bounce builds *elasticity*—the ability to stretch out and then rebound to normal shape.

Side-to-Side Squat

This move begins to take the squat deeper, preparing for the Full Squat. It compresses knees the way you do in a full squat, but it does them one at a time. In the process, it provides a great stretch for the groin and hamstrings.

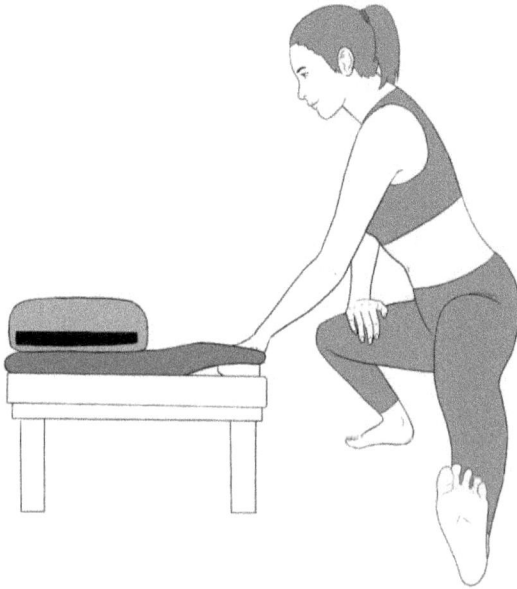

To do the Side-to-Side Squat:

1. Squat down over your right foot.

2. Toes of left foot come into the air as the left leg straightens, so right foot is flat on the ground as you squat over it, and left foot is on its heel.

3. Right hand is on your knee, so you can use it to help press yourself up again.

4. Left is on the bench for balance, or on left leg for a deeper stretch.

5. Lean forward slightly to reduce weight on the legs, then squat to the other side.

6. Stay as low as you can as you move from one side to the other.

Bench Asanas

The bench enables these asanas in ways that no other support–system can. And they're important for sitting well, so it's nice to include them in every session, whether as part of the warm up or at the end.

Leaning Vajrasana (sitting on your heels)

Leaning Vajrasana stretches the thighs near the knee joints, warming up the legs so they can be brought in close for a cross-legged sitting position.

In Vajrasana, you kneel on something soft, then lower your backside onto your heels—if your knee flexibility lets you go that far. If you can't get all the way down, there can be a fair amount of pressure on your knees as the weight of your body pushes you down.

One way to relieve that pressure is to go into Child Pose, where you fold forward and relax with your head on your arms or on the ground. Most everyone can do that pose, even if Vajrasana is out of reach.

But at the same time, Child Pose does little to increase your ability to sit in Vajrasana, because *nothing* is pushing you down.

Another way to relieve the pressure is to put a Yoga Block between your legs, or a bolster on your calves. Then you sit on the support. At the right height, it can be a really comfortable way to sit—but of course, the support means that you can only go down so far. That makes it hard to work your way down to where you are sitting on your heels—if you sit on the support, you don't progress. But if you don't, it's too painful to proceed!

Using the bench makes it possible to find a middle ground, where there is light, manageable pressure that helps you go lower, but not so much that it becomes painful.

A better way is to sit in Vajrasana while taking the weight off your legs. That lets you go as low as possible—but gently, without a lot of pressure forcing you down.

The Initial Position

To do that:

1. Set up a support on the bench.

    *   Lean the small support cushion against the seat cushion. (The best way, as you can use the same set-up for the kneeling back bends.)

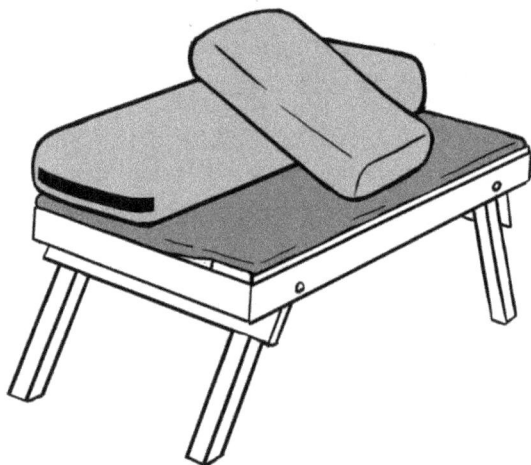

    *   Alternatively, put a couple of Yoga Blocks in the middle of the bench and lean the seat cushion against them. (One will work, but two is better.)

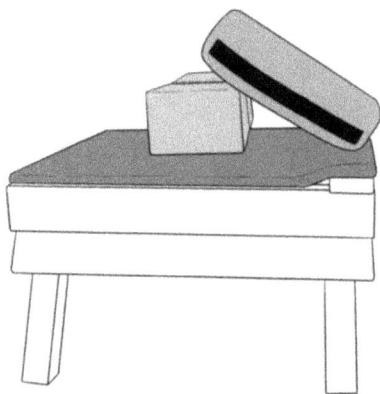

2.   Then kneel in front of the bench, lean forward, and rest your head and chest on the cushion. Put your arms over the cushion, resting them on the other side and hugging the cushion to you, or anywhere else your arms are comfortable.

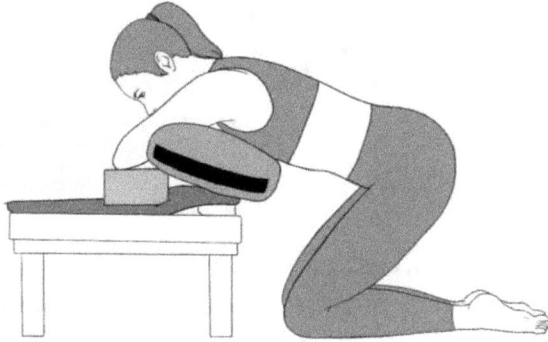

The bench is now taking most of your weight, relieving the pressure on your knees while still allowing you to go as low as your flexibility allows.

Progressing Your Position

Adjust the position as needed. The more upright you are, the more of your body weight is pushing you down. The more horizontal you are, the less pressure there is.

Here is the progression:

1.   **Chest on cushion.**
     Start with the cushion as shown, resting your chest against it and leaning your head or chin on it, depending on where it is.

2.   **Chin on cushion, cushion on edge**.
     As you get more comfortable, move the cushion lower down, so it is against the edge of the bench.

     •   Your chest is still leaning against the cushion, but now the cushion is lower, and leaning against the bench.

- Your chin now rests on the top edge of the cushion.

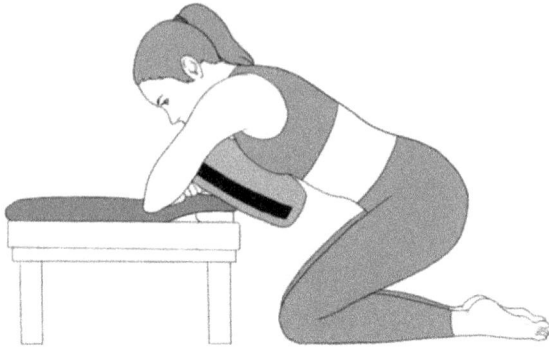

3. **Chin on cushion, cushion on thighs.**
   As you get lower still, keep moving the cushion down to a position where you are comfortably supported until, eventually, the cushion is resting on top of your thighs.

4. **Forehead on seat cushion.**
   Once the cushion is on your thighs, the only way to go lower is to remove it entirely. Your head is very close to the seat cushion, in any case, so it's an easy step. Remove the short square bolster and rest your forehead on the seat cushion. Your forearms are on the bench, in parallel with one hand over the other.

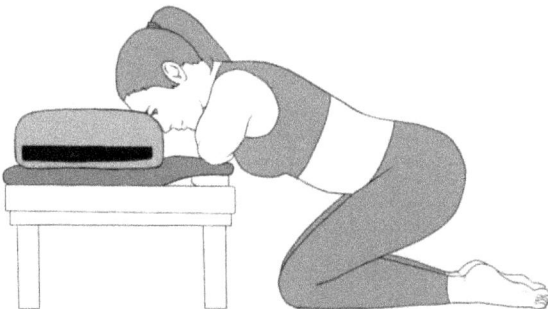

Note:
If your chest is pressing the front of the bench at this point, move your hands to the edge of the bench and rest your chest against them.

5. **Forehead on arms.**

Arms folded on the bench, forehead resting on your arms.

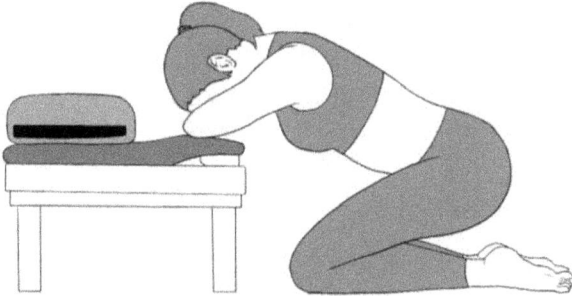

6. **Cupping the chin.**

Elbows on the bench, forearms up with hands cupping your chin. In this position, you are closer to upright, but with much of your upper body weight still supported by your hands.

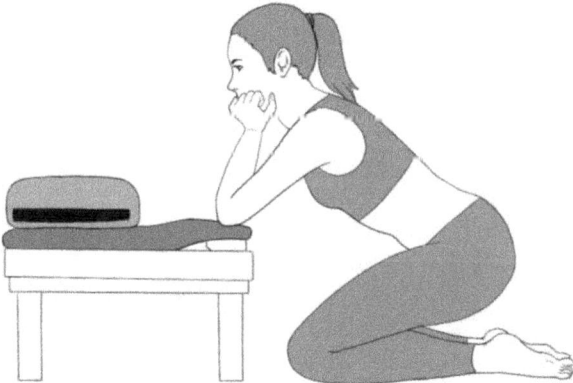

7. **Forearms on bench, body upright.**

Forearms on the bench, with chest raised.

Closer still to an upright position, with even less weight on your hands.

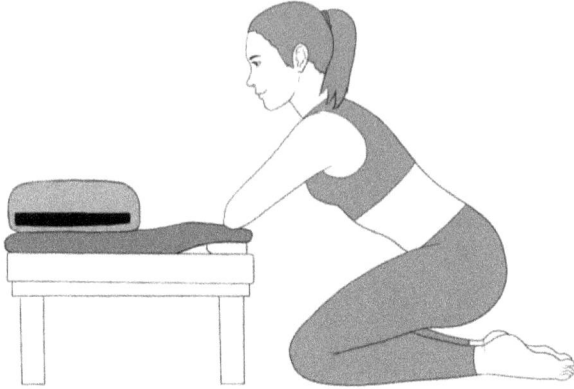

8. **Fully upright, with optional Yoga Blocks.**
   You are no longer leaning on the bench for support. Put a Yoga Block on each side, as needed. Do it as long as you comfortably can, but retreat to an easier position whenever you need to.

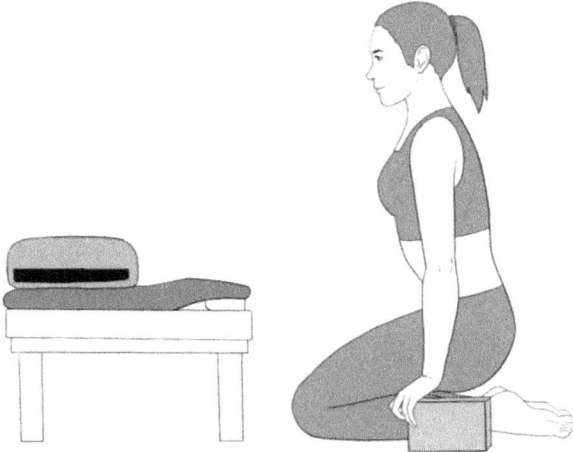

Finishing the Pose

No matter where you are in the progression, it's a good idea to end the practice by sitting upright for a moment. At this point, your legs and knees are warmed up, and not-overtaxed. So they're ready to take the pressure of your body weight (for a short period of time), without undue strain.

Then, by sitting fully upright for a moment or two at the end, you add a little extra motivation—and you also teach your body that it's not so painful to sit that way, once you warm up a little!

After sitting for a moment or two without support (in what is, for you the extreme extension, on this day), place the support cushion on your calves on sit on that. If you're not totally relaxed, put extra cushions or a Yoga Block on top of the support cushion, until you *are* fully relaxed.

Hang out for a while in this position. Notice how your back is perfectly upright. Use the opportunity to meditate for a bit, before moving on.

Bench Bend (Paschimottasana)

For some reason, a sitting-on-the-mat forward bend (*paschimottasana*) is very different from a standing forward bend or the sitting forward bend used to improve sitting flexibility. The latter two seem to depend on flexibility in the hips and glutes, more than the hamstrings.

Paschimottasana, on the other hand, seems to require flexibility in the hamstrings and calves above all else. So I was quite surprised to find that my improved flexibility in other asanas simply did not translate to the sitting forward bend.

In response to that revelation, I began including it as part of my standard Bench Asanas.

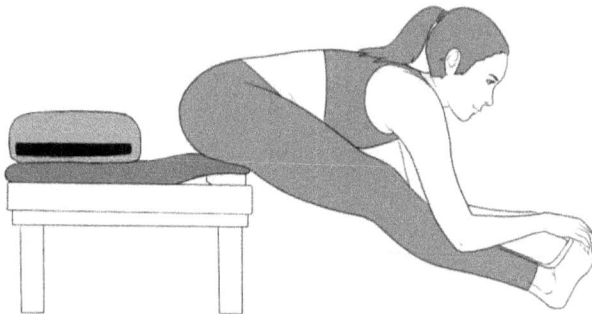

This pose is best done after the standing warmups, which have loosened up the hamstrings and the calves.

To make it easier, put a Yoga block on each side and support your upper body with your hands. If you are just starting out, you may even want to put your hands on the edge of the bench.

As with other forward bends, increase progress by adding some or all of the forward-bending "subtle dynamics" for :

1. Breathe in position, relaxing and moving forward as you exhale. – 2-4 breaths

2. Pulse (inhale while squeezing and relaxing, then exhale with full relaxation) – 2 breaths

    or

    Rock (continuously squeeze and relax while inhaling and exhaling) – 2 breaths

    or

    Alternate those patterns.

3. Maximum squeeze while inhaling, reach forward as far as you can while exhaling, and grab hold.

4. Pull back against resistance as you inhale.

5. Push forward against resistance as you exhale.

6. Pull forward using your arms as you exhale.

7. Back off as far as you need to so you fully relax, and stay there a few breaths.

    Tip:

    To relax and stay in the pose, it can help to support yourself with a Yoga Block on each side of your legs.

If you're flexible enough to reach a couple of cushions placed on your legs, leaning on them can also be a great way to relax in place, as shown on the next page:

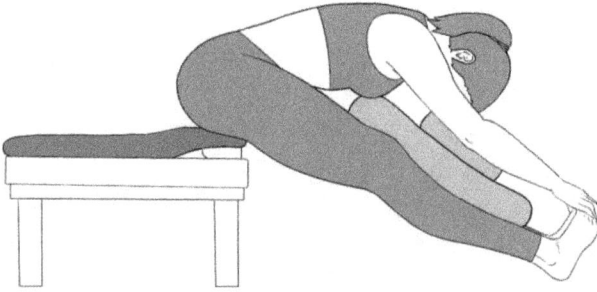

High Camel

In "High Camel", you kneel in front of the bench and place your palms on it behind you, rather than attempting to get your palms all the way down to your heels.

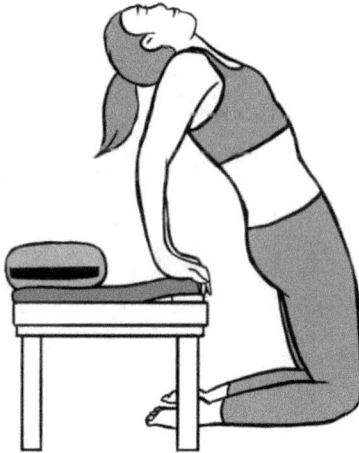

You can put your hands on the front of the bench with palms facing back, or you can put them on the sides of the bench, with palms facing in. (I find the latter position more comfortable.)

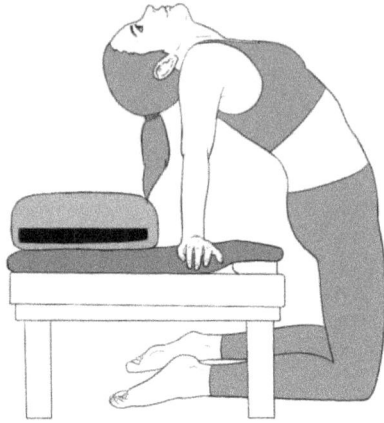

When you're comfortable in High Camel with the bench, you can use a Yoga Block to work your way down to where your hands are on your heels, in the ideal version of the pose.

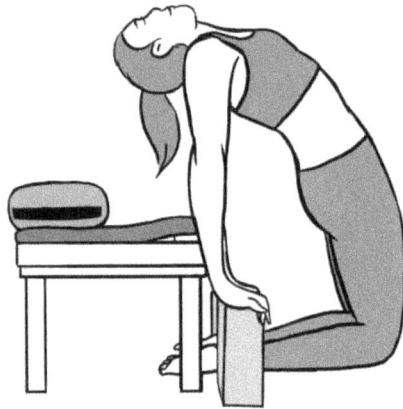

Supported Back Bend (Reclining Warrior)

The Supported Back Bend (aka Supported Warrior in Repose or Supported Reclining Warrior) stretches the full-length of quadriceps muscles (upper thighs), as well as the upper chest and back—all of which need to be flexible to sit upright.

In "Reclining Warrior", if you have difficulty sitting in *Vajrasana* (sitting on your heels), you are likely to lack the thigh-flexibility needed to lower your back to the ground. Without the bench, the best you can do is lean back and brace yourself with your hands on the floor behind you.

Leaning backward in that position does help to stretch the thighs, but it doesn't produce the kind of back bend that Reclining Warrior promotes, and it is often difficult to get into either of those positions, or maintain them for very long.

To make it easier, you can lean backward onto the bench with cushions placed on it.

Note:

I learned this stretch from Vivekadcvi in the Ananda Raja Yoga program. She encouraged putting as many bolsters behind you as you need for support, but a stack that was tall enough for me to use kept falling over! I eventually, put a cushion on a chair—which she then pointed out to the class as a good way to do things. Of course, the back of the chair kept getting in the way—but the bench solves that problem!

The most comfortable cushion-arrangement I have found is to lean a short square bolster against the seat cushion. That arrangement produces an angled support that is exceptionally comfortable—one that even a highly inflexible person can generally reach. You can then relax in that position for an extended period of time to get an advantageous stretch for the back, as well as the thighs.

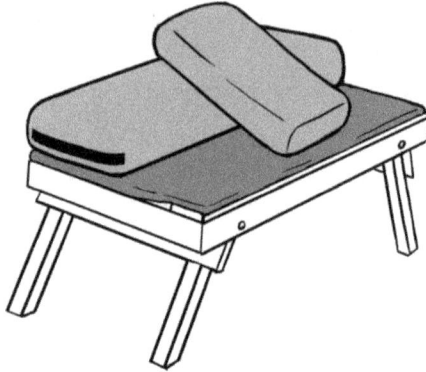

A similar arrangement that comes close to that level of comfort is created by placing a Yoga Block in the middle of the bench, and leaning the seat cushion lengthwise against it. It's not as tall as the first arrangement, but it provides a soft, angled surface to lean on.

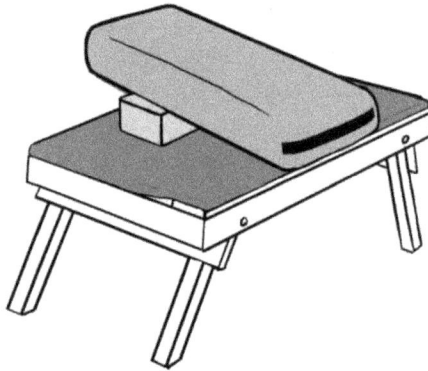

To get the equivalent height from a stack of cushions on the floor, there is a strong likelihood that cushions will move around as you lean back onto them, making it difficult to achieve the desired goal. But with the bench, only the Seat Cushion and an additional rectangular support cushion or Yoga Block are required—and they all stay in place when you lean back!

Follow this sequence. Rest for a bit at each stage, before moving to the next step in the progression. Get into the best position you can manage, stay there a while (breathing!), and then come out of it.

1. Start in High Camel.
   You want your hands at the front of the bench, so you can lower

yourself by bending your elbows.

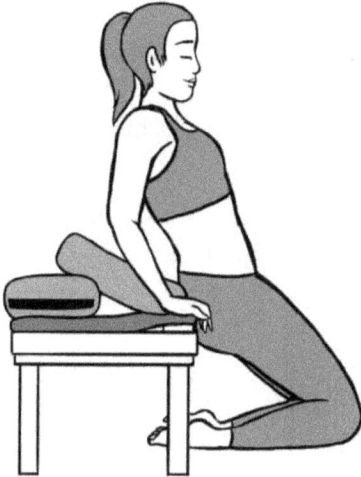

Tip:

To keep your elbows from sliding forward, it can be helpful to grab the base cushion.

2. From there, lower yourself until your elbows are resting on the seat cushion.

    This position stretches your quadriceps. Rest here a while, supported on your elbows, before progressing to the next step.

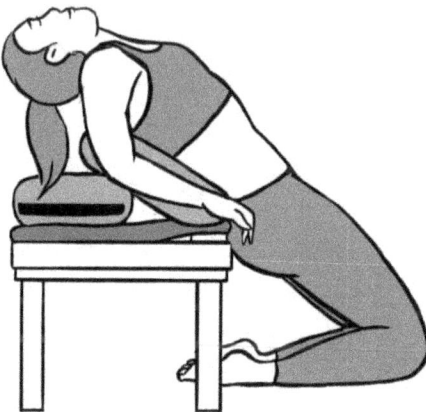

3. Slide your elbows forward, off the seat cushion. This move lowers your back until it is resting on the leaning cushion.

   Elbows can be on the bench, but there is no weight on them.

4. With your back fully supported by the cushions, put your arms out to the sides.

   This movement increases the arch in your back, and gives your upper chest and front of the shoulders a great stretch, as well. (Here, the position is shown with the long bolster leaning against a Yoga Block.)

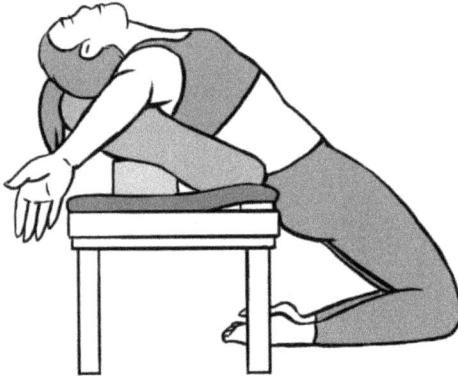

5. To maximize the arch in your back, put your arms over your head and drop them behind you.

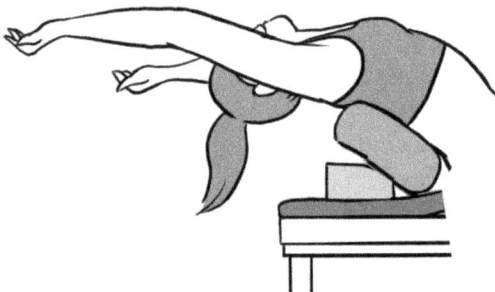

Of course, there are other back-bending poses in Yoga, but the Supported Warrior pose has advantages over most of them when it comes to stretching your back:

o   **Cobra Pose,** where you lift your head and upper back with minimal assistance from your arms, is great for strengthening the back in exactly the way you need it strengthened to sit comfortably. (We'll talk more about that later.) But while it *promotes* back strength, it is also *limited* by back strength—you can only hold it for as long as your back holds out, and your back has quite a bit more flex than your muscles can produce. So while Cobra Pose is beneficial, it doesn't stretch the back as much as Supported Warrior.

o   **Upward Dog,** where you straighten your arms and lift your hips off the ground, does much more to arch your back over its full range of motion. But it can be held only so long as your arm and shoulder strength hold out. So it is as much a strengthening pose for your arms and shoulders as it is a stretching pose for your back.

o   **Bow Pose,** where you lie on your stomach, grasp your ankles, and pull on them as you press your feet away from you, is great for stretching the shoulders, as well as arching the back. The pose can be difficult to get into, and it can be hard to hold, but in addition to stretching the back, the fact that it stretches the shoulders means that your ability to stretch the back is limited by your shoulder flexibility, and your ability to hold the pose is limited by your arm strength.

The point of it all is that while the other back-bend asanas all serve important purposes, none of them let you recline in a fully relaxed position that *really* stretches the back.

The Reclining Warrior pose is the only one that lets you do that, but only does so when you are flexible enough to reach the final position.

Using the bench for support lets you relax the back and stretch it—giving your *quadriceps* (upper thigh muscles) one heck of a stretch, in the bargain.

This is the opposite of the Back Bend, so it makes a nice balancing pose. And with legs warmed up, you'll have the most success with it at this point in the sequence.

Sitting Strength Exercises

This is a bonus section. These exercises do not necessarily require the bench. But as long as I'm telling you how to develop the *flexibility* you need to sit for meditation, I might as well tell you how to develop the *strength* you need.

I call these the *sit strengtheners*.

As an added plus, these short, simple exercises really get your energy flowing! That makes them an ideal prelude for energy-based meditation.

To "sit strong", the areas that need to be strengthened are:

○   Neck

○   Upper Back (shoulder blades)

○   Upper Back (arching)

○   Abdominals

○   Psoas

I've thrown in a few extra strengtheners, just because they're easy to do. They don't take long, and they build health. But most of the strengtheners are devoted to the areas indicated above.

Chest and Shoulders

High-Row Shoulder-Pull Isometric

To keep the shoulders from slumping, the muscles at the front of the shoulders need to be elongated, and the muscles that pull the shoulder blades together need to be strong.

The shoulder flexibility you need is promoted by the Bow pose. The upper back strength is developed with the "High Row".

Using weights and pulleys, you would keep your hands at shoulder level, start with them extended out in front of you, and pull them back to your shoulders, using weight to add resistance.

Using the bench, you can perform a similar exercise by bending forward, grasping the edge of the bench as wide as you can, and pulling your elbows upward against the resistance created by the bench.

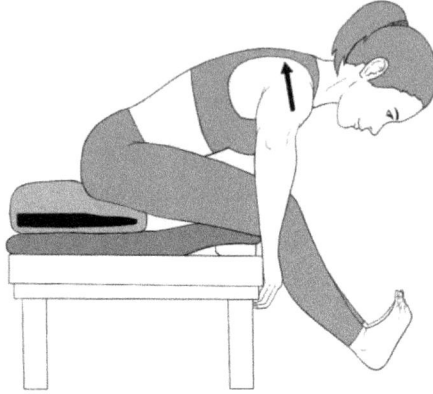

Make sure your legs are straight, with heels on the ground and toes up. (That foot position lets you straighten your legs.) The backs of your knees should be pressing on the bench, so that as you pull upward, you are pulling against your whole body, rather than just the bench (which will lift upward without your weight on it).

With this exercise, your muscles are working, but nothing actually moves. Unlike weights, which travel a certain distance as you exercise, there is no change in distance when you perform this exercise, so it is known as an *isometric* exercise (*iso*, same, and *metric*, distance).

Chest Press

This one doesn't contribute much to posture. But it makes you look better, and it's a good way to balance the High Row exercise you just did.

1. Hold your arms straight out in front, at chest level.
2. Press palms of hands together as you exhale, as hard as you can.

Arm Press

Like the Chest Press, this one doesn't contribute to posture. It's an old Charles Atlas exercise that just "feels right" at this point in the proceedings.

1. Make a fist. Hold it front of your stomach, palm up.
2. Place the palm of your other hand on top of your wrist.
3. Take a deep breath.
4. As you exhale, curl your fist upward (biceps) while resisting with your other arm (triceps).
5. Repeat on the other side.

Upper Back

In the previous section, you warmed up the back muscles. This exercise and the next one will give the back some concentrated attention. For this one, you are focusing attention on the muscles that lift the upper back, isolating them, and strengthening them.

You may know of the standard deadlift, where you use your back muscles to lift a heavy weight from below your knees to your waist. We'll talk about what they do to understand the goal. Then we'll discuss a safer version. However you do it, it is critical for strengthening the back muscles needed to achieve and maintain an upright posture.

What Weight Lifters Do

When done with weights, this exercise is done standing with a barbell across your upper back. (The barbell by itself is sufficient for most. There are no other weights on it.) Or you can do it while placing your fingertips behind your ears, so the only weight you are lifting is the weight of your arms and head.

> Note:
> I'm not recommending that exercise at this point. I just want you to know how it is done.

With a barbell across your upper back, you bend forward at the hips until your torso is parallel to the ground. Then you lift your upper back while keeping your lower back in place, more or less parallel to the ground. When you lower your head, your back rounds. When you lift it, your back arches.

It's a small movement, in which your shoulders move a matter of inches. But it strengthens the back right where you need it to be strong to hold yourself upright.

Weight Lifter's Sitting Version

Done sitting, you bend over and rest your chest (or belly!) on your knees, then lift your chest and shoulders upward while keeping your belly and lower back in the same position.

With your arms hanging down alongside your legs, the only weight you are lifting is your chest, shoulders, and head. To add a few pounds, put your finger tips behind your ears.

To add a couple of pounds more, you can extend your arms straight out in front of you, but that gets awkward—and it tends to work the rear *deltoid* muscles at the back of the shoulders, more than the back muscle you really need.

At this point, a weightlifter will put a barbell across their upper back to increase resistance. But in a moment you'll learn how to do an isometric instead, which is safer.

Cobra Pose

The yoga *Cobra Pose* also exercises the upper back muscle. And that is the *real* reason for doing it. (It's not about flexibility. There is very little flexibility in the upper back!)

In the Cobra Pose, you lie face down on the ground, and then lift your head and upper back, *without* using your arms to press upward. It's the very same muscle, and it's the right one to strengthen. It's just more effective to use the Sitting Isometric, next.

Upper Back Isometric

Sitting has the additional advantage that it lets you do the *Upper Back Isometric* I recommend. This exercise is more effective than the Cobra Pose, because you're working against greater resistance. And it's safer than using weights, as there is no undue strain on your lower back.

> *Note:*
> It is possible to experience cramps, however. That is the result of your body tensing, in reaction to a small pain in a muscle it is not used to using. Fortunately, it is possible to relieve cramps quickly! See the section Handling Cramps and Spasms, that comes later.

To do the exercise:

1. Sit, lean forward, then bend down and grab your feet.

2. If you're thin and flexible, you can do it with knees together. Otherwise, spreading your knees makes it easier to go lower.

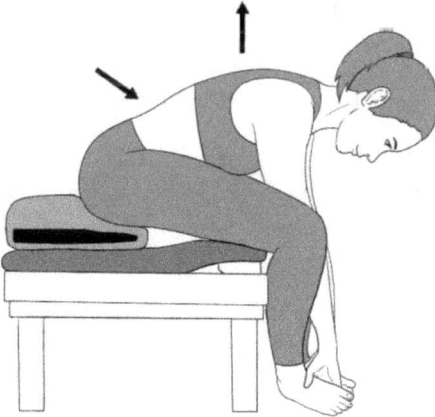

3. As an alternative, you can wrap your arms under your legs, as shown on the next page.

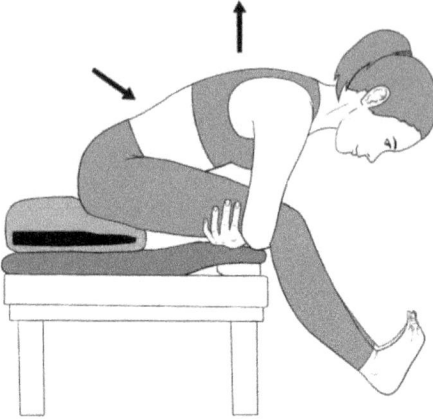

4. If you really need to, grab your shins as far down as you can reach.

5. Take a deep breath.

6. As you exhale, press your belly into your thighs and lift upward with your shoulders, resisting the movement with your arms.

   - With this movement, your lower back will be arched, your chest will be expanded, and your upper back will be doing the work.

7. When you're done exhaling, release the pressure.

Note:

If you have been doing the Advanced Super Enhancements for the bending movements, you have already been doing this exercise in various positions. Here, we are focusing on the exercise itself, without making it part of a bending sequence.

Lower Back and Shoulders

Lower Back Isometric (aka "Deadlift")

The full Deadlift exercise performed by weight lifters exercises the muscles of the lower back. That's an important exercise for core strength. We're going to do one that is perhaps not quite as effective, but which is much safer, which makes it a good choice if you have yet to develop the muscles in that region.

The Lower Back Isometric targets the third section of the back that needs to be strong.

- The first section was the muscles between the shoulder blades that pull the shoulders back, coupled with the muscles that pull them down (shoulder muscles, the *lats* at the sides of the back, and the muscle just underneath the shoulder blades).

- The second section was the mid-back muscle that holds the chest upright over the lower back.

- Now we're focused on the muscles of the lower back, that pull the torso upright over the pelvis.

You can do it with one knee up, or with both feet on the floor.

To do it with one knee up:

1. Start by sitting with one knee up on the bench.

2. Clasp your hands around your shins, or wrap your outside wrist around your shin and grab that wrist with your inside hand. (If your right knee is up, your right arm is your outside arm. Wrap

your right wrist around the shin and grasp it with your left hand.)

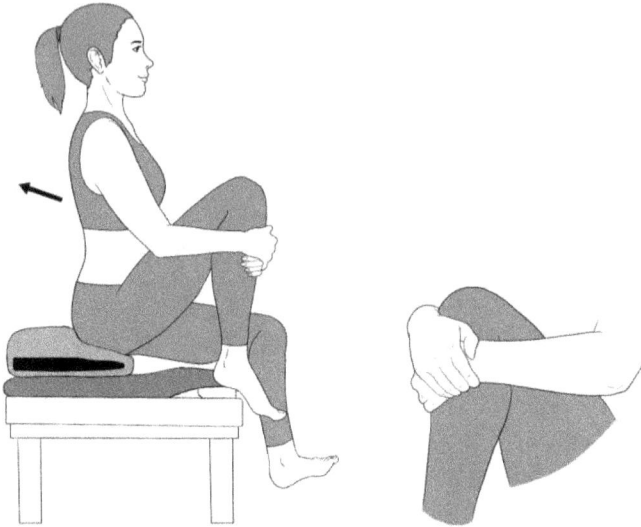

3. Arch your back, and pull backward, resisting the movement with your arms.

The important part is that your back is arched and your back muscles are working. Your arms then provide resistance in one of two ways:

a. **Your arms are straight**.
    To straighten them, your foot and shin need to be pushed away from you and you need to be leaning back a bit. Once you get in position, your arms aren't working very much at all.

b. **Your arms are bent**.
    In this position, your arms are bent at right angles, with your elbows by your sides. Your foot and shin are in close to your body, and you're sitting upright. Your biceps are working in this position, so you tone your arms at the same time. (The good news is that the biceps muscles are at their strongest when the arms are bent at right angles.)

An even better way to do it is with both feet on the floor:

1. Extend your legs with heels on the floor and toes up, so the backs of your knees are pressing on the bench.

2. Grasp the edge of the bench, straighten your arms, and use your lower back muscles to pull back and up.

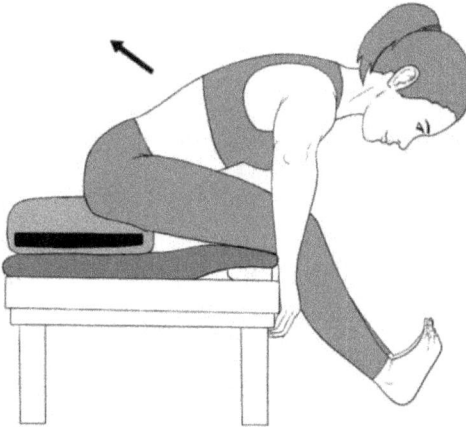

This position is very much like a standard deadlift, but you are doing an isometric, rather than lifting a heavy weight.

Upright Shoulder Pull

This exercise expands chest, promotes good posture. (If nothing else, you feel what it's like!) It also strengthens the *trapezius* muscle that connects the neck and shoulders.

1. Sit on the edge of the bench and grasp the edge.

2. As you exhale, pull straight up with straight arms, giving it everything you have.

Delt Press

The *delts* (deltoids) are the muscles that lift your arms to the sides. They run from the tip of the shoulder down the outside of the arm. Anytime you are doing something that involves having it your arms at shoulder height, it helps to have strong deltoids.

To exercise them:

1. Sit with your knees apart, at the edges of the bench.

- You can sit with both feet on the ground, or with one foot up in Half Tibetan pose.
- You can even sit with both feet up, in either Easy Pose or Full Tibetan, where the feet are lower than your thighs.

2. Make fists with your hands.

3. Sit up tall and place your fists inside your thighs, with the back of your fists touching the thighs.

4. Take a deep breath.

5. As you exhale, push your fists outward against your thighs, as hard as you can.

Hips, Groin, and Psoas

Psoas Isometric

The *psoas* (*soh-az*) are the muscles that connect the upper thighs to the spine. They join to each side of the spine, about a third of the way up, and actually run *through* the hips, to connect to the leg bones.

Most people that work on their fitness these days know that the abdominal *crunch* (where you lie on your back and lift your shoulders towards the ceiling) is recommended because it isolates the abdominal muscles, *without* involving the psoas.

A lot of the sit ups done in the past, with feet held in place, were found to exercise the psoas more than the abdominals. To fix that problem, fitness gurus came up with the crunch.

But the psoas muscles turn out to be *vital* for good posture. When your posture is really good, your middle and upper back are upright and vertical, with your head balanced over them. But your lower back is different: It has a slight curve to the back, in what Gokhale calls the "J" spine in her TEDx Talk on "primal posture".

It is the psoas muscles that create that J-spine—especially when you're sitting. So strong psoas are important!

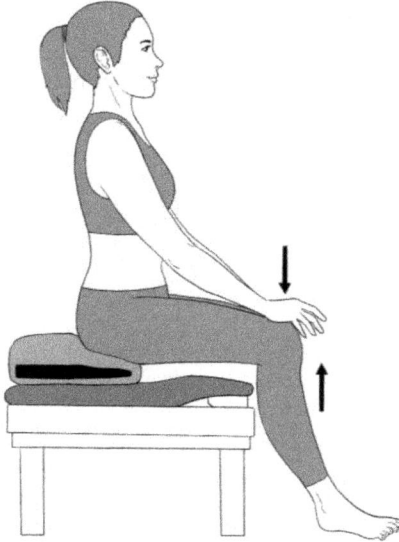

To exercise the psoas isometrically, start by sitting with your knees in line with your hips.

Then:

1. Put your hands on your knees, with arms straight.
2. Inhale.
3. As you exhale, pull your knees upward as hard as you can, against the resistance of your arms.
4. When you're done exhaling, release the tension.

Double-Leg Psoas/Groin Isometric

This exercise works the psoas in combination with the groin, to develop strength in the direction the muscles are used when sitting cross-legged.

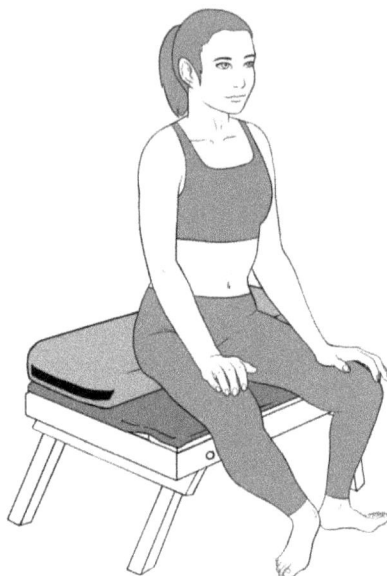

To do it:

1. Spread your knees while sitting on the bench.
2. Lift your knees, resisting the movement with straight arms.

Half Butterfly Isometric

The Half Butterfly is an even more effective way to work the psoas and groin muscles in the exact direction that strength is needed when sitting cross-legged.

To do it:

1. Put one foot up on the bench in Half Tibetan or Half Lotus position
2. Put your hand on that knee with the arm as straight as possible, as in the Double-Leg version.

3. Attempt to lift the knee while resisting its upward movement with your arm.

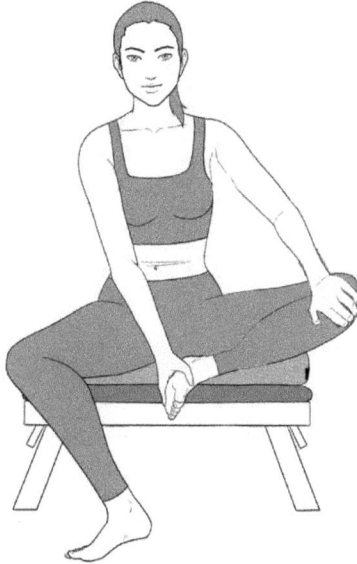

Full Butterfly Isometric

If your flexibility doesn't let you get your knee low enough to straighten your arm, the Full Butterfly position may work better for you. In that position, grasp your ankles and resist the upward movement of your knees with your elbows.

You can also grasp your feet, but only if you keep them pressed to the floor. To do that, you can grasp the middle of the foot, or you can cup your hands around your toes and pull your feet *inward*, toward your body.

Many people make the mistake of grabbing the foot under the toes, and then pulling like mad in an attempt to get lower. That puts an unnecessary strain on the ankle joints, so I recommend grabbing the lower legs instead, just above the ankles. (There is nothing wrong with grabbing the foot though, if you do it right.)

In fact, there is a sequence of useful hand positions you can use:

1.   Grasping the ankles, elbow presses on knee.

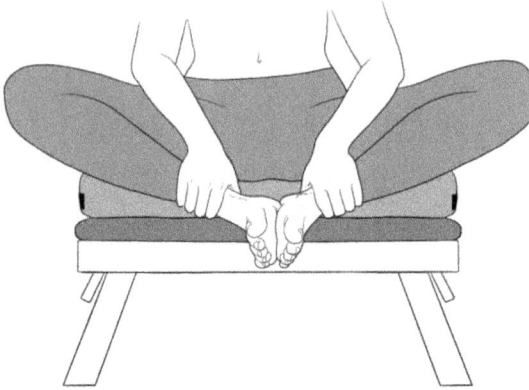

2.   **Grasping the mid-foot.**
     Here the thumbs are inside the arch and fingers wrap around the instep.

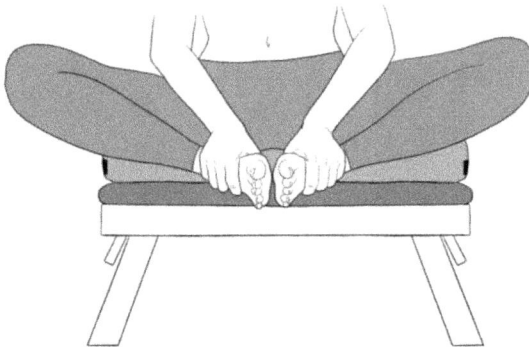

3.   **Fingers curled under the mid-foot.**
     Here the fingers are on the feet, but the palms are on the instep and the thumbs are in the arch of the foot. (The fingers are not under

the toes.)

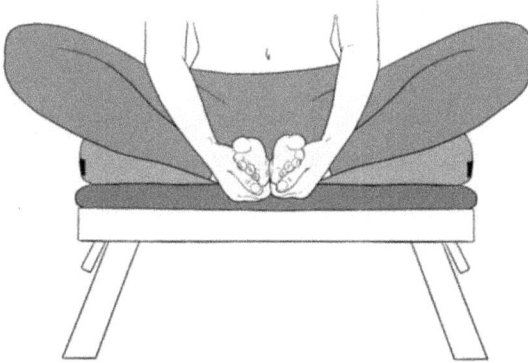

4. **Yoga-interlace around the *front* of the toes.**

    Here, you use the Yoga Interlace finger position to wrap your fingers around the front of the toes. This is a good position to use when you want to pull your torso forward. When you do, you are pulling straight back against the feet (rather than pulling the toes upward, which does you no good).

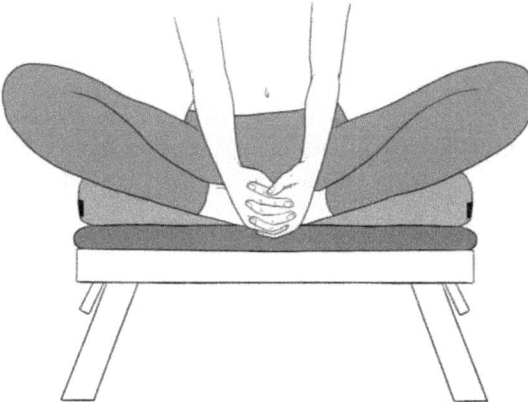

Abdominals

Bench Boat

This is a good abdominal toner and conditioner. Get into position, then squeeze the muscles you're using as you exhale, giving it everything you have.

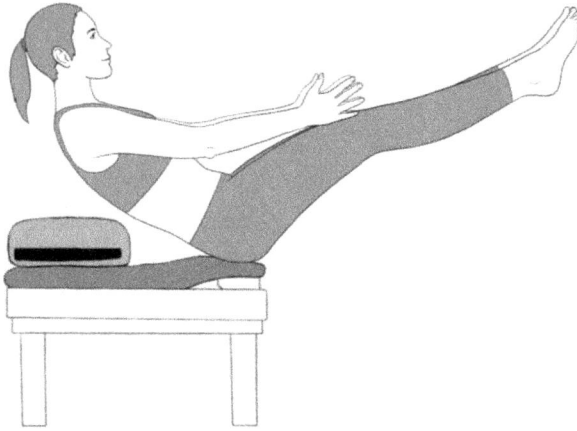

Bench Bridge

This short exercise mostly works your backside, but does a little for the abdominals as well. But strong glutes are important for posture (not to mention good looking), so I am including this exercise.

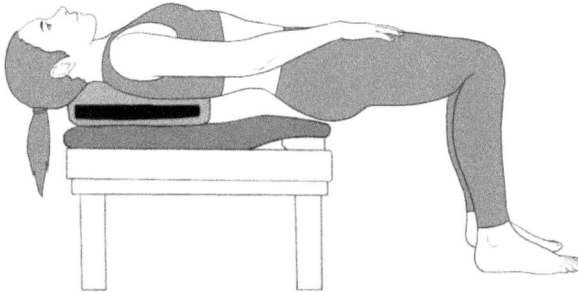

To do the Bench Bridge:

1. Sit on the edge of the bench.

2. Support your weight with your hands as you shift a little farther forward.

3. Lean back until your shoulders are on the seat cushion.

4. Lift your buttocks , so your torso is level with your knees. (If your legs are short, move forward and put your shoulders on the edge of the bench.)

Standard Yoga Asanas

Many of the standard asanas involve standing, doing back bends, or sitting on the floor. The Yoga Bench provides assistance in each of those areas.

For Meditating *Between* Asanas

When you have a standard Yoga practice, one of things that can make it even better is to meditate between asanas, or between a series. For example, I typically meditate after each of the series described earlier.

But there are other kinds of series, as well. Perhaps you do the *Surya Namaskar* (Sun Salutation) series. Or you might do a series of forward bends and the reverse back bends. Or perhaps you have other sets of asanas that move nicely from one to the next, *Vinyasa Flow* style.

After each series, I encourage you to sit for a moment, experience the internal energy flows they release, and bask in the warm glow of your efforts! You may find that adding those meditations makes your practice that much more enjoyable.

> *Note:*
> In addition to a standard "meditation", you can also perform "subtle energy dynamics" like the standard Yoga mudras and bandhas, or the so-subtle-no-one-knows-you're-doing-them versions described in Volume 3 of this series. You can even do subtle pranayama practices without alerting people next to you. All of those practices invigorate the body while at the same time producing a sense of joy and higher connection.

In a Yoga class, you're encouraged to rest in Child Pose when you need to take a break. That's fine for your physical body, but it does little to put you in the kind of posture where you can *feel* the energy flows and *enjoy* the benefits of your exertion. For that, you need an upright, *meditative* posture.

Of course, as any weightlifter knows, it is important to take a rest after you have stressed your body. That gives your body a chance to recover from the exertion, so it is ready for the next one. That rest makes those efforts you just finished more productive, and it lets you recover the energy you need for your *next* series.

If you're comfortable sitting on the floor, that's terrific. You can take meditation breaks whenever you want! But if you're not totally comfortable on the floor, those "breaks" are simply an additional stress! In that case, although the breaks are intended for relaxation and meditation, they wind up taxing your body even further.

I have personally seen a new martial arts student who, through no fault of his own, was unable to sit upright on the floor! He was the victim of living in the West, where a lifetime of sitting in chairs had virtually eradicated all flexibility in his hips.

It was impossible not to feel sorry for him. Unable to bring his knees to the ground or to tilt his pelvis enough to bring his back over the tripod created by his thighs, he sat there with ankles crossed, knees up in the air, leaning backward with a rounded back—all the while struggling to keep from falling over backwards.

Having been in that exact position myself, I knew that his back was getting sore, and that the *psoas* muscles that connect the upper thighs to the spine were straining to keep him from falling backward. In less than a minute, critical muscles were *aching*—all while sitting in a position that was supposed to allow him to relax, meditate, and recover from the warm up exercises.

Needless to say, he didn't last long. How could he? Instead of having an intermittent series of exertions, every moment he spent in class was a strenuous, energy-draining effort!

But, today: Ta da! *Super bench* rides to the rescue! With the bench present, anyone who can sit in a chair can sit and meditate, relax, and recover, whether they are practicing Yoga or martial arts.

The practice of meditating between each series, then, coupled with the bench, can put a strong Yoga practice within reach of *everyone*.

For Teachers

In time, practitioners may even reach the point where the bench is totally superfluous. And that would be grand! Experienced Yoga practitioners are already there. So anyone who has had a regular practice for three years or more probably has no need for the bench, and may well be teaching.

In that case, in addition to encouraging the practice of meditating between each series of asanas, I encourage you to think of your students! Providing benches for them can make it possible for them to experience the *kind* of practice you enjoy, even if it is at a much lower level, initially.

And because they *can* do the practice at a lower level, it becomes possible for them to gradually *increase* that level, until one day they, too, can dispense with the bench.

For Standing Asanas

For standing asanas that involve bending or lunging, the bench itself can act as a support that is slightly taller than a Yoga Block in its tallest orientation.

For a taller support, the base pad can be removed, or the edge pulled back, and a Yoga Block can be placed on the bench. The block can be placed on the base pad, as well. If the pad is soft, the block is securely ensconced in the pad.

The three different orientations of the Yoga Block then provide three additional levels of support at 4 inches, 6 inches, and 9 inches above the bench.

When standing upright, as in the Yoga tree pose, even a tall Yoga Block placed on the bench will be lower than the fingertips of most adult users. So some other accessory is needed to use it as a hand balance.

Tree Pose

This is one pose for which the back of a normal chair is an advantage, rather than something that gets in the way. Of course, you can always do what people did before they used chairs, and touch a wall, tree, or bit of furniture for balance.

However, by simply standing *next* to the bench with your lower leg contacting it, that slight assist can help to stabilize you until you find your balance. Then, over time, you develop the strength and sense of balance to maintain the pose on your own.

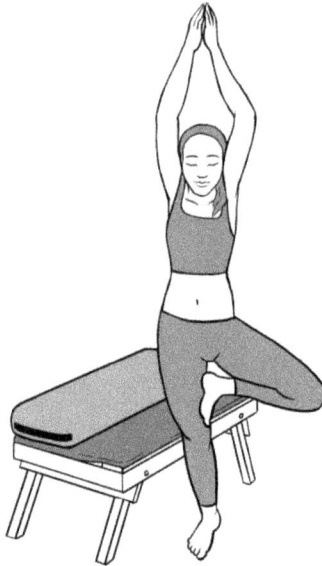

Standing Dive

This is one of my favorite poses using the bench. When both hands are out in front, it's like you're standing on one leg and diving, A block on the bench helps you keep your balance while developing strength.

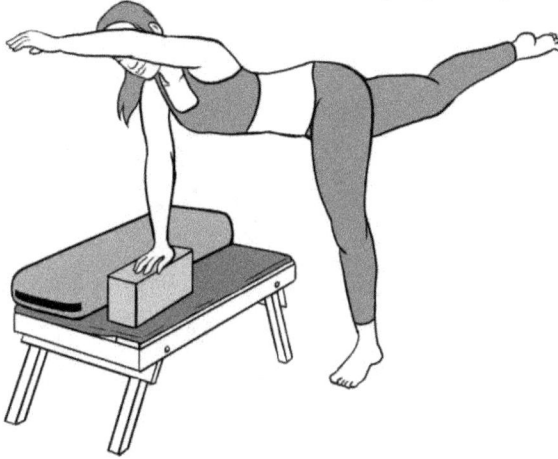

Warrior Lunge

Put both hands up, palms facing each other for a pure Warrior Lunge, or use the bench for balance while you develop the strength for this pose. (A chair is too tall to be of much use here, but the bench height is perfect.)

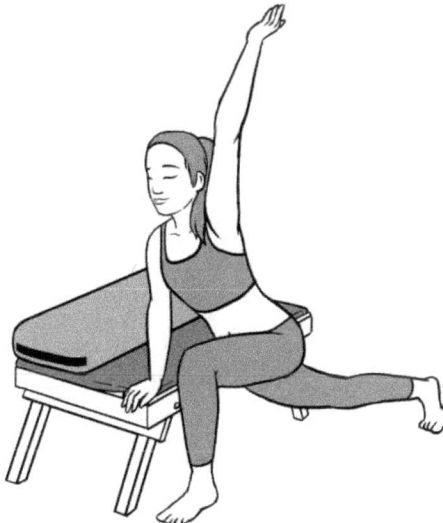

Supported Triangle

Using the bench and optional Yoga Block, you can get support at the exact height you need.

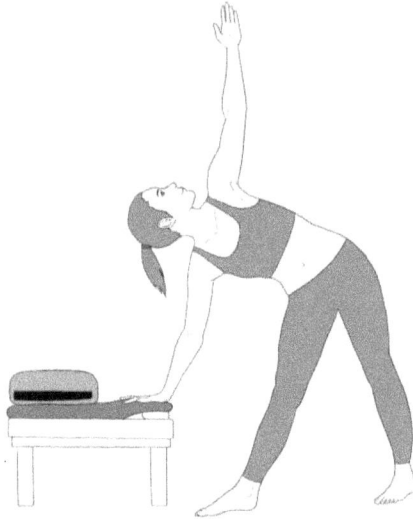

In medium-height orientation, the Yoga Block is at just about the same height as a chair. But unlike a chair, it is easier to go a couple of steps lower, with your arm still locked out for support.

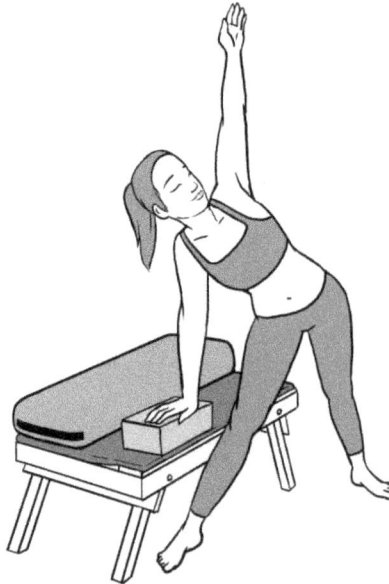

For Floor Asanas

Getting older is a pain in the *tuckas*. (I'll say it again: Don't do it! It's a mistake! But does anyone ever listen. No....)

Even simple things get hard, when you're older. Those things can also be hard when you're injured, or you simply lack strength. That's why staying "young" is a matter of staying strong, flexible, and energetic! So that's one reason you're doing Yoga of any kind, and a major reason you have the bench.

The other important reasons are to experience internal energy flows and to connect with the power and wisdom of the "universe energy", which goes by many names, including "god". But there is only so much I have room for in this short volume, so I'll have to leave with that hopefully-tantalizing hint.

Okay. Back to the main message. Let's see... Where was I? Oh yeah, I remember. We were talking about using the bench for asanas done on the floor. Let's start with the simplest thing: getting up and down.

Getting Up and Down

Simply using the bench as part of your Yoga practice makes it easier to get up and down:

- From a standing position, you can put a hand on it to lower yourself.

- From a sitting position, you can put both hands on the edge of the bench and lower yourself to the floor. (If you want, you can push yourself back up again. But that's an exercise. It's called a *dip*. But let's ignore the fact that it might actually be good for you. Let's just focus on the fact that it can make things *easier*.)

- When it's time to get back up again, you can put one or both hands on the bench to steady yourself or take some of the weight.

In other words, simply using the bench to get up and down helps to make Yoga more approachable for many who would otherwise experience great difficulty.

High Bridge

A nice back arch, made easier by the bench.

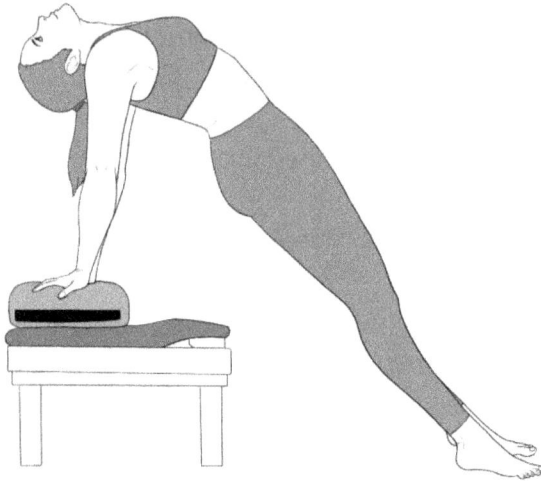

Supported Janusirasana

In this pose, you tuck one foot in to the inside of your thigh and stretch forward over the straight leg. You can bend forward while sitting on the bench with one foot up, but that leaves you without a lot of support. This version lets you rest on the bench until you're flexible enough to go lower.

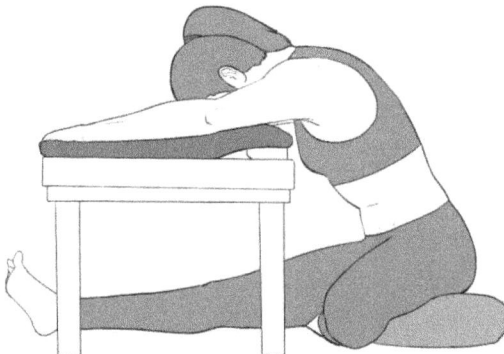

Half Butterfly

On the floor, you do the Half Butterfly with one leg straight, and with the other foot tucked in to your inner thigh. That works great—if you have the hip-flexibility needed to sit upright in that position.

With the bench, you don't need any special flexibility. You put one foot on the bench, and the other rests on the floor.

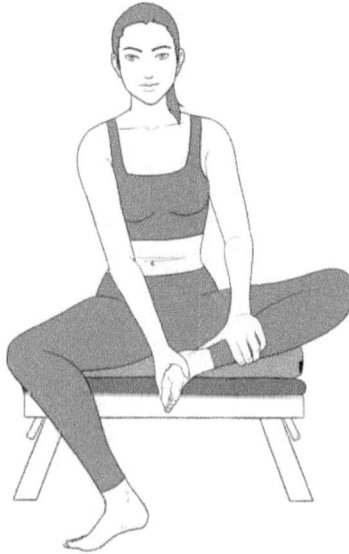

This position is very similar to the Half Tibetan pose. The only difference is that the ankle is bent and the foot is in the middle of your seated position, directly in line with the groin, rather than moved over so it is under your thigh.

If the foot that is supposed to be tucked onto the bench won't quite get there, use a Yoga Block Footstool to move it as far up from the floor as you can. (You can also do that in a chair. But the difference is that the last step (foot up on the seat) is easy on the bench, and much more difficult in a chair.)

Once you are in the Half Butterfly position, you can either simply breathe and relax, or do the Dynamic Subtle Energy Sequence for an even better stretch. As with the sitting forward bends, do the movements three ways:

1. Push your upper knee towards the bench.
2. Bend straight forward, with your other knee straight in front.
3. Bend over the upper foot and thigh next to it, with the knee at an angle out to the side.

Full Butterfly

This is the standard Butterfly pose, with the soles of your feet together and tucked in as close as you can get them to your groin.

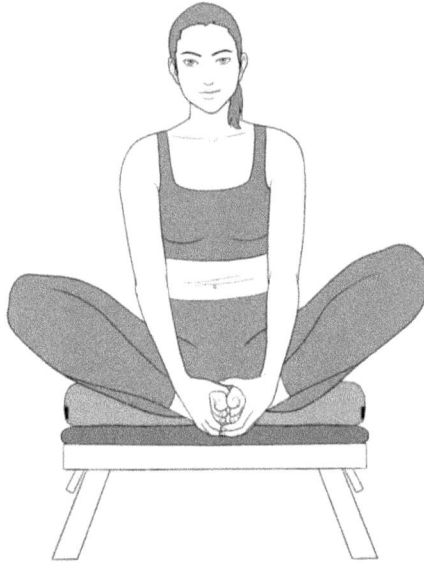

As with the Half Butterfly, you can use the Yoga Block Footstool, as needed, to gradually move your feet up to that position.

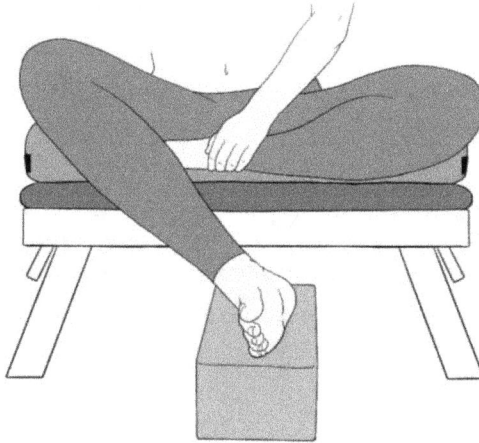

Once there, there are two kinds of movement patterns:

1. Knees to the bench

2. Bending forward

In each position, you either breathe and relax as you press (knees down or body forward), or you can do the movement sequence.

Don't Flap!

One thing I do *not* recommend is "flapping your knees like a butterfly". I've seen people told to do that move in both martial arts programs and Yoga studios. My considered opinion is that it is remarkably ineffective, and risks injury.

If your groin is generally flexible, and you're simply a bit tight at the moment, that move isn't too bad. It serves to increase blood flow to the area and loosens you up. So people who have already developed flexibility can possibly be forgiven for thinking it's a good idea.

If you are *not* already flexible, you can't flap far enough to do yourself any good. And if you try to flap harder, so your knees make a sound when they hit the ground, it is all the more likely that you will create a minor tear as you pull the groin muscle.

The truth is that the "flap your wings" style of Butterfly Pose is another great *test* of your flexibility. If your flexibility is good, you'll be able to hit the ground and make a sound. And the closer you can get, the more flexible you are.

But trying to *improve* your flexibility with that move is pretty much a fool's errand.

Side Bend

In my warm up sequence, I do a side bend without worrying about putting an arm overhead. But if you're used to the standard Yoga asana, here's the bench version:

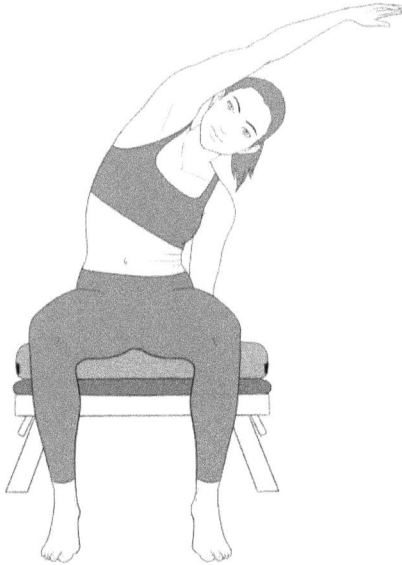

Supported Wheel

The wheel pose, where you arch the back with hands and feet on the ground, produces a long, backward arch that is good for the spine. But it takes a lot of strength to push yourself up into that position and strength to maintain it—until you achieve enough flexibility that your arms and legs are effectively "locked out" at full extension.

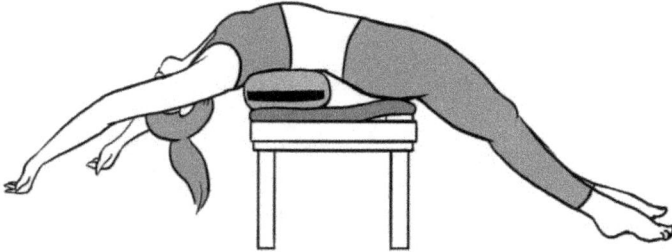

Once you achieve that level of flexibility, the pose becomes much easier to maintain. In fact, only about as much effort is needed as it takes to stand—because each part of the arms and legs is stacked on top of the part below it so, as with standing, the bones are taking the weight of the body, rather than the muscles.

Until you reach that point, however, it is your muscles that are doing the work, and they tire quickly. As in other forms of Chair Yoga, you can lie down with your back on the bench, feet on the floor and arms in the air behind you.

You can then simply rest in that high-arched position, getting the benefit of the back bend without muscular effort, or you can reach down to the ground and push yourself up from that higher position, which requires much less effort than is needed when pushing upward from the ground.

Iyengar Back Arch

B.K.S. Iyengar uses this position in his Chair Yoga practice. It's like the Supported Reclining Warrior, except that you sit on a cushion to make the position even more comfortable.

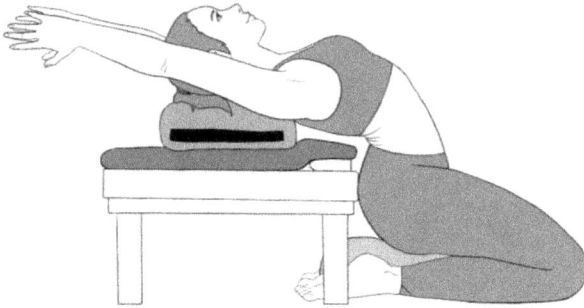

For a higher support, lean the cushion against a Yoga Block.

Plow Pose (Halasana)

For *Plow Pose*, you are supposed to lie on your back and then lift your legs over your hand, placing your feet on the ground behind you. It is an excellent inversion, but to be performed properly, it requires flexibility in the back, hamstrings, and *gluteus maximus* (backside).

Lacking the required flexibility, many people wind up with their feet dangling in the air, or they strain their necks attempting to go far enough to reach a supported position.

Placing your feet on a Yoga Block can help, but it is difficult to get the block into the right position. Or you can use a chair, turned sideways so the back of the chair isn't in the way. You can also purchase a *Halasana Bench* designed specifically for that asana, but while it is helpful, it represents a significant investment for a piece of furniture that has a single use, and no other purpose.

The meditation bench gives you an alternative. You can place your feet on the bench or on cushions placed on it. (Since it is fairly large, it is easy to find with your feet.) Or you can stack up a cushion or two on the bench and rest your shins on the cushion.

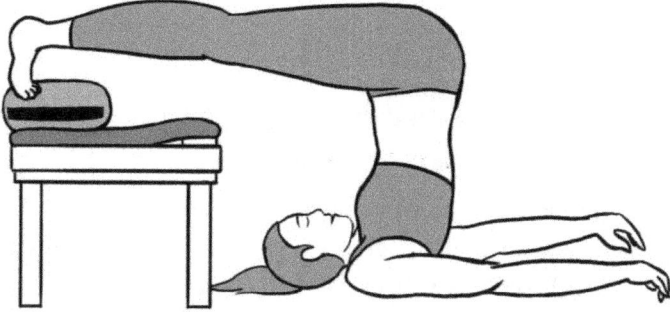

You can then relax in the pose for long enough to develop the flexibility you need in the hamstrings, glutes (backside), and back.

Go higher by putting a Yoga Block under the seat cushion.

Go lower by:

1.   Putting shins on the cushion.

2.   Putting feet on the bench.

3.   Putting shins on the bench.

Eventually, you may arrive at the maximum position, where you get your feet to the floor, (preferably with a cushion under your back to protect your neck). But there is plenty of benefit to be had before then.

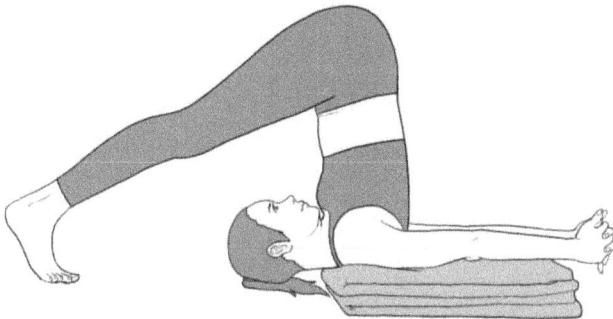

Peacock Pose (Mayurasana)

Peacock is a physically demanding, muscle-strengthening pose I could do when I was a teenager. It has been out of reach for many a year now, but the bench makes it possible to re-approach that position.

Difficult to Do on the Floor

Done on the floor, the pose is difficult for several reasons:

○   **Wrists hurt**
It is hard to put your palms on the floor with your fingers pointing back at you. It puts a lot of pressure on the wrists and fingers. Try it! You'll see. (If you don't, you're young. Good for you! Don't change. :__)

○   **Nose bangs the floor**
You start in a kneeling position, with your knees spread. Then you put your palms on the floor. Now, you are supposed to "walk your feet back" until your legs are extended behind you.

There is just one problem with that strategy. Until your legs *are* fully extended, they don't act as a counter-balance. So, as you begin to lean forward, you essentially fall towards the floor, head first.

Ideally, you'll want to rest your forehead on the floor, rather than your nose, but either way your face is approaching the floor on what, over the years, has become a rather uncomfortable speed!

It's a chicken-and-egg problem, you see. You need to have your legs extended to keep your head off the floor, but your head needs to be at or near the floor to extend them!

○   **Gut is in the way**
As a 6-foot tall, 150-lb string bean of a teenager, nothing got in the way of my elbows. I could bring them close together into the pit of my stomach, creating the pivot point (or *fulcrum*) for my body.

Sadly, those days are long gone. Height hasn't changed, but girth has been enhanced considerably. So what was once quite easy has become a lot more difficult.

One way to solve the problem of the gut is to connect your elbows with a strap. Placed just above the elbows, it gives your body a fulcrum to rest your body on without requiring your elbows to be adjacent.

Another way to solve the problem is to be strong! The web is rife with photos of people doing Peacock Pose with their elbows at their sides! Of course, these are all young, strong, super-fit people. It's great to *be* that strong. The problem is to *develop* that strength.

The bench can help.

Using the Bench

Peacock Pose isn't exactly *easy*, with the bench. But it's a lot eas*ier*.

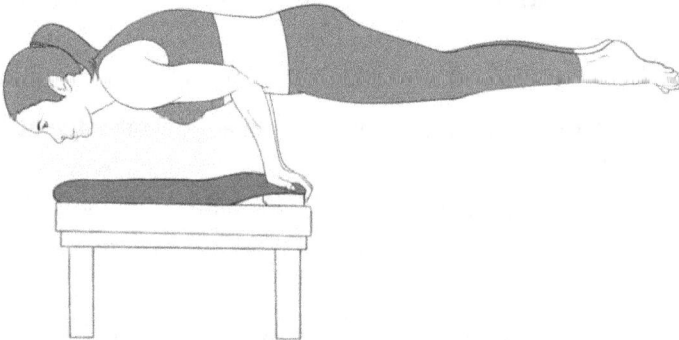

In the first place, rather than having your wrists on the floor, you can have them on the edge of the bench, on the Foot Rail. That position takes the pressure off your fingers, which reduces the pressure on the wrists.

This is the same principle that gymnasts use when they learn handstand. They'll be the first to tell you that a handstand on the floor is hard on the wrists. To acquire a sense of balance and the strength to maintain it, they learn with mini-parallel bars (called *parallettes*) that are about 6 inches off the ground. Grasping those bars takes away the pressure on their wrists.

Secondly, the bench keeps your nose off the floor!

There are two ways to get into the Peacock position on the bench: Shoulders First, and Hips First.

To do the **Hips First** variation:

1. **Stand facing the bench.**
   Start by standing in front of the bench, facing it, with the seat cushion in place.

2. **Squat and place your hands.**
   Squat until you can place your palms on the foot rail, with your fingers curled over the front edge of the bench. (If the base pad is in place, lift it slightly to get your hand under it.)

3. **Place your thumbs.**
   Your thumbs can curl over the edge of the bench, in line with your fingers. Or they can stay on top of the foot rail, pointing to the edges of the bench.

4. **Lean forward until your shoulders are resting on the seat cushion.**
   You may "fall forward" a bit, but your nose won't be in any danger.

   - **To make it easier, rest your knees on the edge of the bench.** With most of your body weight taken by your hands and knees, it's a lot easier to get your shoulders down to the cushion without "falling". (To make it more comfortable, keep the base pad in place when you do this pose.)

   - **To make it easier still, add the short square bolster.** The extra height of the support cushion makes it easy to get your shoulders down to the cushion. Your head will then be too high to lift your legs, but you can work your legs back, get a sense of the position, and begin developing the strength and flexibility you need to perform this difficult pose.

5. **Adjust your hands.**
   With the weight of your upper torso resting on the seat cushion, and the weight of your lower torso taken by your knees on the bench and/or feet on the ground, it is easy to adjust the position of your hands and elbows.

6. **Walk your feet back.**

   It's now easy to do, as the weight of your upper body is resting on the bench.

7. **Lift your legs and your shoulders.**

   As you lift your legs, lift your shoulders off of the seat cushion. Ideally, you'll get to where your body is parallel to the ground. Work up to it!

To do the **Shoulders First** variation:

1. **Kneel in front of the bench.**

2. **Rest your shoulders on the seat cushion.**

   Lean forward with your hands on the bench until your shoulders are supported by the cushion.

3. **Extend your legs and place your hands.**

   Extending your legs moves your hips up, making room for your hands and arms.

   It is now easy to put them into position.

4. **Move your legs farther back.**

5. **Lift legs and shoulders.**

Personally, I find the Shoulders First variation easier to get into, but for some reason it is harder on my wrists and hands. The Hips First version seems to be easier on my wrists, but fear of falling (despite the cushion!) makes it harder to get into.

> *Note:*
> Another way to do this pose is to rest your hips on the bench, as Allison Ray Jeraci does in this great Yoga International article, Mayurasana Made Easier: Use a Chair. That way of doing it gives you a sense of the position, and helps to develop the strength needed for the full version.

Build Great Posture ("Posture Plan")

If you have been using the bench for a while, you may have discovered that, while you need flexibility in your legs to sit cross-legged, sitting comfortably *at all*—even in a chair—is about *posture*.

Just by sitting on the bench, your neuromuscular system is learning the point of balance for your spine, head, and shoulders that produces maximum comfort—a balance that it will *automatically* work to maintain throughout the day.

And, as you sit, you are strengthening the muscles you need to maintain that balance. So the longer you sit, the stronger you get!

So far, you've learned how to use the bench for sitting and meditating, for sitting asanas, and for standard asanas. And have learned a variety of exercises that build the *many* muscles that go into maintaining your posture. (Perhaps more than you knew!)

Now it's time to put them together into a schedule that, over time, will create the *strength* and *flexibility* you need to maintain a comfortable back in any circumstances.

Ideally, spend 20 minutes a day on this practice, and you'll restore your strength and flexibility in no time!

Identify Your Goal

First, let's understand what *great* posture is. The picture on the next page shows what many would consider to be "good" posture.

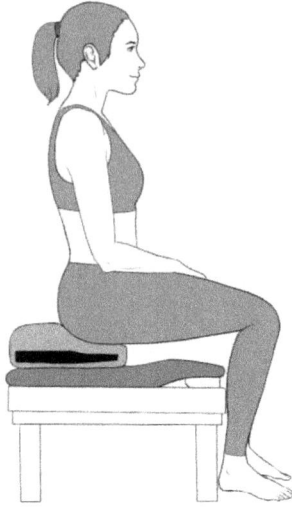

Many people would look at that posture and say that she is sitting well. But there are subtle issues that will cause stress over time.

Note that her shoulder's aren't *quite* over her hips. That's because her head is slightly forward of where it needs to be. Because her head is forward, her torso has to lean back slightly to compensate.

Here, on the other hand, is *great* posture:

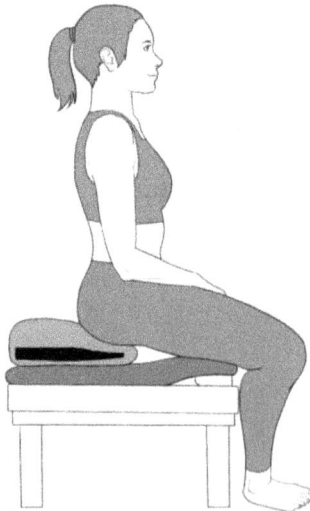

Here, the chin is pulled back a bit, so the ears are directly over the shoulders. The shoulders, in turn, are directly over the hip joints.

Her legs are out to the corners of the bench, as well, which lowers her knees. That lowering, in turn, allows for the vital *pelvic tilt* that produces a vertical alignment of the spine.

The slightly increased tilt of the pelvis can be discerned in the drawing, along with the increased arch in the lower back. (It may be somewhat disconcerting to realize that a "straight, upright spine" is created by protruding buttocks. Nevertheless, it is the case!)

Create a Three-Session Sequence

Now that we know what we're going for, we're going to a design a schedule that works for you! If you practice 3 days a week, this schedule is a natural. If you practice 6 or 7 days a week, you can do this schedule twice!

If you meditate, you'll find that these practices lead naturally into your meditation practice. If you don't, you can do these practices while watching TV or conversing with your roommates or spouse. (Visitors may not understand, but people you live with should!)

Pick Three Sitting-Flexibility Asanas

To start, pick the most difficult pose you can sit in for each leg—in reasonable comfort—from the following list. Then pick a second and third most difficult, ideally from different groups:

- o   Advanced Group
  - Lotus
  - Tailor
  - Half Lotus
  - Quarter Lotus
- o   Intermediate Group
  - Half Tailor
  - Perfect Pose

- Tibetan Pose
- Easy Pose

   o Basic Group
- Half Tibetan, 2nd leg wide
- Half Tibetan, 2nd leg straight ahead

   o Beginner Group
- Both feet on floor, legs wide
- Both feet on floor, legs together

For each pose, remember that you can use a Yoga Block as a foot rest to gradually increase the level of difficulty.

At the time of writing, the poses I've selected for my personal practice are:

1. Quarter Lotus
2. Perfect Pose
3. Half Tibetan (plus Half Tailor, 'cuz I need it)

Now then, for scheduling, on the first day of your three-day sequence, choose the easiest pose in your list. On day two, choose the 2nd most difficult. And on day three, choose your most difficult pose.

For each pose, go through the full movement sequence! You may find that you progress faster than you ever thought possible!

You can then do each pose on its scheduled day. It works as-is if you have three-day-a week practice, or you can do it twice and take a day off for a 7-day schedule.

Additional Extras

Supported Warrior in Repose

This standard asana is very important for your sitting flexibility—much more important than it is commonly given credit for.

It loosens the typically-tight muscles running across the top of the chest and the front of the shoulders. Because they're tight, they make your head and shoulders slump forward, putting strain on your neck and on your back.

The Supported Warrior with arms out to the sides is ideal for stretching and loosening those muscles. It needs to be part of your posture-building plan.

This stretch can be taxing, so it is probably best to do on your easiest day.

Cobra Pose / Sitting Strength

The standard Cobra Pose asana builds the strength in the upper back—the most critical muscle for good posture. On your medium-effort day, do that pose if nothing else.

For more comprehensive strengthening, do as many of the Sitting Strength exercises as you can.

Leaning Vajrasana

The ability to sit cross-legged in comfort requires flexibility in the quadriceps muscles that run along the tops of the thigh, along with the ability to compress the knee. That way your lower leg can bend to where it is nearly parallel with the upper leg. That flexibility lets you bring your foot close enough to your body to achieve a crossed-leg position.

Leaning Vajrasana is a great way to achieve that flexibility. Do it first, the day you sit in your most difficult positions, to help you warm up for the positions to come.

Subtle Energy Squeezing Series

Each of the full-blown exercises described earlier can also be done in a more subtle manner. When done that way, someone looking on may not even notice that you are doing anything. Nevertheless, the exercises are effective—both for strengthening muscles and for stimulating energy flows.

The series can then be followed by the subtle internal contractions that define the Yoga *mudras* and *bandhas*—subjects that will be dealt with at length in Volume 3 of this series.

Squeezing Sequences

To do the exercises, focus on the muscle in question and squeeze it. Hold the tension for an exhalation or so, and then release it. Instead of an all-out, muscle-shaking, body-quivering tension that affects an entire area, you are isolating a specific muscle and giving it a more mild, internal tension.

Individual Muscle Squeeze

Take a breath or two between each squeeze. Be aware of the internal sensations, and enjoy them.

Working from top to bottom, the squeezing exercises are:

1. **Back of the neck.** (smaller version of Neck Isotonic)
2. **Squeeze shoulder blades** together (small version of Shoulder Pull)
3. **Mid-back** (smaller version of Upper Back Isotonic)
4. **Diaphragm**
5. **Lower back** (smaller version of Deadlift)
6. **Abdominals**
7. **Psoas** (upper thighs at the hip joints)
8. **Groin** muscles
9. **Squeeze-and-Relax** any area of the body that needs strengthening or healing

Segmented Squeeze

Once you know the individual muscles, you begin working them in groups. Here is a sequence that squeezes them in combinations, working from the top down:

1. **Neck/Head** (mostly the neck, but can also include face, eyes, gums, etc.)
2. **Chest / Upper Back / Upper Arms**
3. **Abs / Lower Back / Fists and Forearms**
4. **Hips / Upper Legs**
5. **Lower Legs and Feet**

As always, many different combinations and sequences are possible. Let your spirit be your guide!

Breath Patterns

There are several breathing patterns you can use for the muscle-squeezing sequences. Here is a progression from simple to complex. In all cases, breathe slowly with a full Yogic breath:

o   Squeeze while exhaling and relax while inhaling.

o   Squeeze while inhaling and relax while exhaling.

o   A multiple-breath sequence.
    Start by inhaling and holding, then exhaling and relaxing. **Then:**

a.   Inhale – hold – exhale and squeeze the muscles in an area.

b.   Inhale feeling energy entering and gathering at the chest and head
    – hold – exhale directing it to the area.

c.   Inhale – hold – exhale and relax, be aware of sensations.

    Repeat the sequence as many times as you like for a given area, before moving to the next.

Benefits of the Squeezing Series

As simple as the squeezing sequence is, it provides a lot of benefits:

○ Strength

○ Relaxation

○ Lymphatic Drainage

○ Bone Growth

○ Energization

○ Healing

Strength

Squeezing a muscle strengthens it, and promotes muscle growth—without going to a gym, without special equipment, and without lifting weights.

It may not be quite as effective as those activities, but it is a *lot* more effective than doing nothing.

> *Note:*
> As mentioned earlier, Charles Atlas promoted such "dynamic tension" exercises for strength training and body building in the early 1900's. At around the same time, Yogananda was teaching a series of "Energization Exercises" that were very similar. Regardless which came first, the technique is undoubtedly effective. (But I would still love to know! Who gets the credit?)

Relaxation

The Science Direct website has a great PDF, Learn more about Progressive muscle relaxation that details the history and science of muscle tension as a prelude to relaxation, beginning with its origins in 1905.

Yoga classes often use that practice at the beginning of *Savasana*, where you lay on your back and fully relax. To promote that relaxation, you are often instructed to tense and release sections of the body, working in a sequence from the top down or bottom up, and finishing by tensing the entire body.

Again, one has to wonder: Which came first? Did Yoga incorporate tension and relaxation into the program after scientific research demonstrated its unique benefits? Or was the original scientific research given direction by some experience with Yoga?

I suspect the former, because it is highly unlikely that any Western scientist was practicing Yoga in 1905, given a lack of classes and teachers.

But the latter is not *impossible*. A lot of underground "psychic" investigation was going on at the time, and even Tantra and Kundalini were becoming known to the West, in at least some circles. So it is entirely possible that a scientist was inspired in some way by practices that were passed on from one person to another.

Either way, we know that squeezing a muscle causes the entire area of the body to relax more fully and completely—especially, when there are muscles that have been *unconsciously* tensed. Consciously squeezing and relaxing the muscle builds your awareness of it, making it possible to feel it when it has tensed, so you can relax it.

Lymphatic Drainage

The *lymph system* carries the white blood cells that combat disease. It also carries away toxins and metabolic wastes. It also absorbs fatty acids from the intestinal tract and puts them into the blood stream.

Unlike the blood stream, the lymph system doesn't have a heart muscle that provides a pumping action. In essence, the lymph system is like a series of small tubes (like soda straws) joined together, with a one-way valve at the end of each tube.

When the muscles around the valve are compressed, lymph is pushed upward through the valve to the next tube. From there, it can move forward, but not back.

In short, muscle activity is *necessary* for the lymph system to function. Without it, waste builds up as if the garbage-collectors were on strike. The immune function is impaired, as well, as though the drivers of the EMT (emergency medical technician) vehicles were *also* on strike.

The squeezing exercises therefore do a lot to improve body function and immune system operation.

Learn more:

- Lymphatic System: Facts, Functions, and Diseases
- Lymphatic System (Wikipedia)

Bone Growth

The people selling you supplements for your bones rarely tell you one important fact: A bone only grows in response to *muscular stress*. When a muscle pulls on the bone, it grows. Otherwise, it doesn't.

The lack of weight training and other forms of resistance exercise is therefore the main reason that women tend to be more prone to *osteoporosis* (weak bones that break in a fall), along with the fact that, historically, men tended to be doing the more physically demanding jobs.

The squeezing exercises have the advantage that they put at least *some* stress on the bones, without requiring any weight to do it.

Of course, resistance exercise with weight is probably even more effective. In that case, the squeezing exercises are, at the very least, a lot better than nothing.

On the other hand, it may be that the squeezing exercises are *better* for bone growth, because they pull on the bone from all directions, in a way that doesn't cause muscular fatigue. (Which means they can be done every day.)

The ability to stress a bone from multiple angles and the ability to do the exercises every day suggests that, even if they are not quite as effective as *free weights* (dumbbells or kettlebells, for example), they are probably more effective than machines that force you to move in a single direction.

On the other hand, machines where you pull on a cable are probably in the middle somewhere. But are they more effective than muscle-squeezing, or less effective?

Research would be beneficial to answer the question. But, in the meantime, it is helpful to know that the squeezing exercises do promote bone growth, to at least some degree.

Energization

In addition to the increased blood flow and oxygen that gets to the area, Dr. Tennant claims that exercising a muscle pushes electrons from the outer "muscle batteries" into the cells underneath the muscles.

Of course, it may simply be the inflow of oxygen that is responsible for the extra electrons. (The internal cellular batteries—the *mitochondria*—are re-charged by a process that burns fatty acids to release electrons from oxygen.)

Either way, the fact remains that additional electrons are made available to the cells underneath the muscles—cells that include organ tissues, tendons, ligaments, and bones.

The additional electrons provide, in a word, *energy*. It's an energy you feel, right after doing the exercise. So the squeezing exercises can also be called *energization exercises*.

In fact, that is exactly what Yogananda called the versions he taught! (I believe the versions I describe here are even more effective. They *feel* that way from my personal experience, at least. But this is another area where good research would be valuable.)

Healing

Squeezing and relaxing for the purpose of healing is an effective practice that Yogananda taught. He called it "Quiver Healing". We wanted the muscles under so much tension that the muscles begin *quivering*.

I have no doubt that squeezing the muscles to that degree is even more effective for healing. In the meantime, know that any kind of squeeze-and-release cycle does promote healing to at least some degree.

As to how it works, we know that squeezing a muscle moves metabolic by-products out of the system through the blood vessels and the lymph. That action clears the way for oxygen and nutrients to arrive and to be integrated into the cell.

That action also energizes the underlying tissues by increasing the number of electrons. If Dr. Tennant is to be believed, the energy required for a cell to replicate itself (which is how it grows and repairs damage) is twice its normal voltage—in other words, twice as many electrons as it normally contains.

So, by increasing lymph drainage, squeezing metabolic by-products out through the veins, increasing the flow of oxygen and nutrients, and by upping the electron count, the muscle squeezing exercises work to promote healing and growth!

The Body Battery

Science is coming to understand more and more that the body—and indeed the universe, from galaxies down to atomic sub particles—are *electrical* in nature. And where there is electricity, there is magnetism. So opportunities for investigating electro-magnetic effects abound!

My "YouTube U" playlist contains a myriad of videos that bring this information to light, including great videos by Wal Thornhill (the Electrical Universe theory), along with other great videos from the Thunderbolts Project and others on plasma theory and the nature of magnetic fields. Those videos have been, in a word, *illuminating*.

Although the chemical model of the body has come to dominate academia for the last 100 years or so, a new, fundamentally *electrical* paradigm is beginning to take hold. One reason for that shift is the all-but-utter failure of the chemical model when it comes to treating "lifestyle diseases" like diabetes, heart disease, and cancer. Another is the way it so frequently overlooks the body's enormous capacity to *heal itself*.

The Body Electric by Dr. Robert Becker does a great job of reviewing the long history of scientific investigation into the electrical properties of the body. It details how, under the right conditions, those properties can be used to stimulate regeneration of missing tissue—up to and including entire limbs.

A later research, Dr. Jerry Tennant, has given a number of talks recorded on video (see the Resources), plus a book (Healing is Voltage). His book does a good job of summarizing more recent information on the subject.

Energy is Electrical

When Dr. Tennant and other scientists measure the voltage of a cell, they are measuring the number of *electrons* it contains. We all know that electricity is energy, and electricity is nothing other than the flow of energy, so it makes sense that the "energy circuits" (*nadis* in Yoga, *meridians* in Tai Chi and acupuncture) are pathways along which electrons flow.

Of course, electrons don't actually move *through* those circuits, the way they might in an electrical circuit. But it is quite possible that electrons in one cell exert pressure on electrons in a neighboring cell. When the electrons in the second cell move away from the first, they would exert more pressure on the electrons in the cell next to it, and so on.

If that is the case (and I hasten to admit that I am speculating), it is possible that a string of cells would exhibit the characteristics of a circuit, and that a lack of electrons in a clump of cells would reduce pressure in that circuit.

Oxygen and Energy

According to Dr. Tennant, the higher the voltage of water, the more oxygen it can contain. On the other hand, he also reports that, inside the cell, it is oxygen that provides the electrons that recharge our tiny cellular batteries—the *mitochondria*.

If both statements are true, then the more energy you have, the more energy you *can* have, because of the increased capacity of the cells to take up oxygen.

On the other hand, it is entirely possible that, in reality, the measurement of "voltage" is simply a measure of how much oxygen the cell has taken up, and therefore how many electrons have been freed for use as energy.

Of course, I am giving an extremely simplistic summary of a very complex chain of internal events. And my understanding is limited! (See the Resources for a PDF that explains the many interactions that make up the energy production and utilization cycles.)

The point here is that the issue is complex! So when a scientist measures voltage in a cell, it's not clear to me what they are actually measuring.

What *is* clear is that oxygen is critical to energy production. (As is water, of course, if only because it enables the Krebs Cycle activity that burns fatty acids to recharge the mitochondria—another great reason to stay hydrated!)

Oxygen is critical to energy production.

Adding Pranayama (3-Part Yogic Breath)

Since oxygen is part of the energy-generation process, deep-breathing pranayama practices can and should be part of the muscle- squeezing exercises!

The principles and practices of pranayama will be covered in depth in Volume 3 of this series. For now, use this version of the *3-part Yogic Breath*, also known as the *Complete Breath*:

1. **When you exhale, exhale fully and completely.**
   The goal is to expel all of the carbon dioxide that has accumulated in your lungs.

2. **When you inhale, expand the abdomen, then the ribs, and finally the chest.**

This is the "Complete Yoga Breath". Pause for a moment at each stage, before going to the next.

There are outward physical versions of this practice, and an even more effective inward "subtle" version that will be covered in Volume 3. But if you focus on expanding each area in turn, you'll get a complete breath.

3. **After you inhale, hold as long as you comfortably can.**
    Don't strain, but do hold the accumulated oxygen in your lungs. This is when the lungs exchange carbon dioxide that has been put into the blood stream by the cells (a by-product of metabolic activity) for the oxygen in the air.

4. **Exhale from the chest, then exhale from the ribs.**
    At each stage, pause and relax. From here, breathe normally to discontinue the practice, or move to the next step to start a new cycle.

5. **Contract the abdominals for a complete exhalation.**
    This is an active movement that begins a new breath. You're no longer simply relaxing and letting air flow out. Instead, you are actively moving it out. That action gets most all of the carbon dioxide out of your lungs, paving the way for a new influx of oxygen.

The Body as a Battery

You can visualize your body as a giant energy circuit. The bottom of the spine is the "negative" pole, where electrons are generated. At the top is the "positive" pole, where they flow to. (And where, as a result, your positive thoughts and positive energy emerge!)

The muscle squeezing exercises help to activate that circuit. In effect, you become a giant battery, with positive energies accumulating at the top, where they are just *itching* to be released into the world.

As the voltage rises, you begin searching for ways to make a positive contribution to the world! And that is how, as a people, we *all* benefit when someone meditates, does Yoga, or exercises.

Your Personal Practice

Handling Cramps and Spasms

This one tip could save you a small fortune in pain medications and muscle braces. (You're welcome!)

When your body feels pain in a muscle, it tends to tense that muscle. Unfortunately, the action of tensing increases the pain, which increases the tension, and so on, in a vicious circle that exercisers know only too well.

Nutritionally, you want to increase your uptake of magnesium and potassium to minimize cramps. But there is an incredibly simple, immediate solution as well: *Work the opposing muscle.*

To relieve a cramp, work the opposing muscle.

What to Do

For example, if you are experiencing a cramp in your back, sit or stand with your hands on your knees (or elbows on a table), and do an *abdominal isometric*—contracting your abdominal muscles in an attempt to push your shoulders to your knees, while resisting that motion with your arms.

You will feel an immediate, slight release of muscle tension. And that is often enough to trigger a release-of-tension cascade that reverses the cramp, where each release/relaxation is slightly bigger than the one before, until the muscle is completely relaxed.

If you've had the spasm for a long time, your neuromuscular system may have begun to build an ingrained pattern that causes the muscle to spasm whenever it feels the slightest stress. In that case, even a massage can trigger it!

If so, then you might need to repeat the isometric. But if what you're experiencing is a muscle spasm, it will definitely work. (I've rarely ever had to do it more than twice, and I've *never* had to do it more than 3 times, personally.)

Why It Works

When you exercise a muscle, the immediate, automatic neuromuscular response is to relax any muscles that oppose its action. It's a built in safeguard that keeps your muscles from working against themselves.

So when you do an abdominal isometric, your back relaxes. When you lift your toes against resistance, your calf relaxes. And so on. So wherever you're feeling a cramp, work the opposing muscle and watch it disappear!

> *Note:*
> I learned about this magical move from a YouTube video created by Dr. Marco. It's based on a reflex-principle that is also used in stretching. I knew about that reflex-principle, but never realized it could be applied to cramps. So I could not be more grateful!

Your Time, Your Way

Perhaps the greatest benefit of a personal practice is that you can spend exactly as much time as you need, exactly where you need it.

My practice focuses on meditation. So while the sequences I perform can generally be done in 20 or 30 minutes, my practice generally takes about an hour!

Some days it is short. Maybe I'm just not "feeling it", so I don't do as much. Or maybe it will be longer than normal. That tends to happen when I get lost in meditation. The energy flows may be so strong, and my sense of communion so powerful, that it takes a while to come out of it. But my practice is just that—*my* practice! It's as long as it needs to be!

Vinyasa/Tantric Flow

One way to build your practice is to focus on *flow*.

Vinyasa Yoga focuses on a smooth flow between postures. That's a great concept. I would also add the concept of movement that is part of Tantra Yoga—something I learned from Shakti Padmini, who teaches in San Francisco's North Bay.

When Shakti Padmini does Yoga, it's like nothing so much as a *dance*. While in a pose, she is moving her body in whatever way her inner feelings are directing her. She's never static for more than a moment. And when she moves to a new pose, it's in a sinewy, dance-y kind of way.

That is a Yoga I can recommend!

Done Tantric-style, there is no fixed pattern of poses. You listen to your inner voice and go where it directs. You feel your body and add any movements it calls for.

The sequences you have learned so far are the things that came to *me*, during *my* practice. They developed over a long time. Feel free to develop your *own* practice, and teach it to others!

My Time, My Way

These days, my practice follows the pattern below. But that practice has changed several times over the last couple of years! I offer this pattern as one that is worth engaging in, but I do not suggest that it is the only possible practice. As always, let your inner spirit be your guide.

Built-In Meditations

Each of the practices after the preliminary meditation are followed by a sitting meditation—generally with internal energy-activation techniques that are covered in subsequent volumes. (For example, I do an extended set of "mini-bandhas" that work like magic to activate internal energy flows. I look forward to sharing them with you.)

When it comes to the meditative pause between segments, the advice that Swami Asanganand gives with respect to Pranayama works beautifully:

When your mind becomes active,
return to your practice.

That advice applies to pranayama, but it *also* applies to every other energy-generation technique described in this series. Because each of them produces the kind of energy flow that precipitates meditation.

I would make a slight change to his advice, however, to make it clear what he means by an "active" mind:

As long as your mind is still,
or is focused in the present,
or is centered on your chosen focus,
remain in meditation.

That covers a lot of ground. But if your chosen focus is feeling the love of your guru, for example, and you are basking in that glow without a lot of extraneous thinking, keep on doing what you're doing! (The same goes for a class, in my book. There is no need to keep following the instructor if you're already where you want to be!)

Practice Outline

Here is the practice I currently follow:

1. **Preliminary meditation**
   A short period of quiet, just to "check in".

2. **Sitting Warmups**

3. **Standing Warmups**

4. **Bench Asanas**

5. **Sitting Strength Exercises**

6. **Pranayama**

7. **Strong Leg Flexibility Asanas**
   Because it is my stronger leg, this is my preferred position for meditation. So this is the "high point" of the practice. I will tend to

stay in meditation longer here than at any other point. I will also tend to meditate after each asana in this series.

8. **Weak Leg Flexibility Asanas**

Although I've already had a great meditation, I'll do as much as I can here. If my weaker leg is feeling up to it (in other words, there is no discomfort), I'll put my stronger leg on top of it and sit in Half Lotus or Perfect Pose.

9. **Closing Meditation**

At this point, I will generally return to my comfortable stronger-leg sitting position. If my weaker leg is feeling comfortable, I may bring it in front of the stronger one, so I'm sitting in Tibetan Pose. But if it gets uncomfortable, I'll put it down again.

In any case, I'll sit for a while longer in a contemplative state. It's a great time to inwardly express gratitude to the teachers and gurus who came before, and to the internal guide who leads me now.

10. **Namaste**.

This is the end of the practice. It's time to acknowledge all those who brought you here, and inwardly express gratitude for their efforts. It's also time to acknowledge your companions on the path. As I learned in my Tantra classes, "Namaste" is the act of acknowledging the divinity in you, seeing it in others, and *recognizing it as one and the same.*

11. **Finishing Sequence**

By this time, legs and back are getting pretty stiff. Time to stand up and go through the 60-second routine that restores fluidity!

Notes:

o *Pranayama* is covered in detail in Volume 3 of this series. My personal practice consists of the 3-Part Yogic Breath with a pause at each stage, Kapalbhati (skull cleansing), and "Nadi Shodana Bhastrika" (a combination-technique I learned from Swami Asanganand).

o The internal energy-activation techniques I use during meditation practice are also described in Volume 3, and taught in person.

Stronger Leg vs. Weaker Leg Asanas

In your practice, you may have two stronger legs, or two weaker ones! The asanas you do and how you do them will therefore depend on your personal level of flexibility.

The Strong Leg and Weak Leg versions of the sitting asanas are demonstrated in a video on the YouTube Bench Yoga Channel. The key differences are these:

1. **Knee Push**

   The knee of the stronger leg goes to the bench easily when the foot is up, and stays there easily. So the Knee Push exercise is not needed. The knee of the weaker leg does not go as easily, and is not as comfortable when in position so, for the weaker leg, I include the Knee Push exercise.

2. **Lower Leg Position for Forward Bend**

   For the Sitting Forward Bend, hip flexibility in my stronger leg lets me get my hands to the ground comfortably. So I flare my leg out to the side. For the weaker leg, hip flexibility is more limited. For that leg, I put my thigh straight out in front of me so I can use it to support my chest, and I will frequently put a hand or fist on my knee to raise the level of support.

3. **Use of Yoga Blocks**

   For the stronger leg, Yoga Blocks aren't needed for the Sitting Forward Bend. I use them only for the Sitting Angled Bend. Even then, they are in their lowest orientation, so fairly soon I may be dispensing with them altogether. For the weaker leg, I use Yoga Blocks for both asanas.

What I Leave Out

Several things described in this book are *not* part of my current practice. For example, at the moment of writing I am not doing the Subtle Energy Squeezing sequences as a distinct practice. Instead, I have folded them into my warm up routines.

Similarly, I am not currently doing the Posture-Building Sequences. During the last couple of years, as the practices got developed and written down, my posture has improved dramatically, and many of those ideas have been folded into my standard practice.

At the moment, I am not doing the Standard Asanas, either. It is possible that I *should* be doing them. But, given that my current practice takes anywhere from 30 minutes to an hour, that is enough, for now. So I offer those asanas for those who are familiar with the standard asanas, and who want to use the bench to help develop their capacity to do them.

I can only say that, at this moment in time, I am not feeling the inward pull that tells me I *need* to do them. My personal goal, after all, is to sit in meditation—in Lotus Pose, one day. So I focus on the techniques that will get me there.

When you get to Volume 3 you'll find *dozens* of energy-flow activation techniques. Time simply does not permit doing them all! So the collection of practices I do regularly tends to change over time. Think of them as a painter's palette. Choose your colors to create the picture you imagine!

Stand By for Evolution!

The point of what I have written in this section is that my practice has evolved. Yours will too. Mine started with 5- and 10-minute meditations. It grew to include sitting flexibility exercises, then strength exercises, until eventually it was taking an hour and half, with meditations.

Then life intervened, and I was back to the 20-minute variety for a while. Then it evolved forward again, in a new direction. Each time I withdrew, it was back to the core of the practice—short meditations. And each time it evolved, it was like adding a new branch to the tree, each branch growing in a new direction towards "sunlight"—the ability to sit longer, sit stronger, and connect better.

I expect that your practice will follow a similar pattern. In the process, your practice will evolve. And you will too.

The Big Picture – The Point of it All

To my mind, the sitting position asanas and the sit strengtheners are the most important part of my practice—except for the *meditation*. After all, the *goal* of Yoga is "union" (or "yoking") with a higher strength and wisdom. The *path* that gets you there is meditation, and a basic *requirement* to take that path is the ability to sit comfortably.

In other words, "to get there from here", you need the ability to be able to sit comfortably!

In fact, in Hindi, the word *asan* means "place where you sit". So the word *asana*, which we commonly translate as "Yoga pose", can equally well be construed to mean "things you do while (and for) sitting".

Actually, it's the same word in both cases: "asan" and "asana" are just different pronunciations, from North and South India, respectively. So how did "asana" ever come to mean anything *but* sitting?

For that matter, what is the purpose of all the *other* Yoga asanas—the ones that develop strength and flexibility, but which don't directly contribute to your ability to sit comfortably?

The answer from gurus and Yoga teachers is that they are intended to keep your body healthy and to keep energy flowing internally. As my martial arts master, steeped in the Buddhist tradition, used to say, "your body is your temple".

In actuality, though, your body is more like your *car*. It is the *vehicle* that takes you down the path towards enlightenment. If your body isn't healthy, and the energy isn't flowing, then meditation is scarcely possible!

And that series of thoughts, believe it or not, takes me to weight training and other forms of exercise. You see, exercise promotes the release of growth hormone. And, in addition to burning fat and building muscle, growth hormone promotes all kinds of healing.

That is its job, you see. It promotes tissue building. So wherever new tissues are needed, whether in a muscle torn down by exercise, or in an organ that needs to work better, growth hormone is the trigger that gets the job done.

For that reason, I think traditional Yoga practice (strenuous as it is!) overlooks important tools in the toolbox of health when it avoids strength training, cardiovascular training, interval training, and other forms of exercise.

Granted, those exercises are not sufficient unto themselves! They need to be balanced by flexibility training and meditation. Nevertheless, they are important for maintaining the vehicle that takes you towards enlightenment!

So I encourage you to consider the Sit Strengtheners and other forms of exercise as part of your "enlightenment practice". Because, when all is said and done, enlightenment is *the whole point* of Yoga.

Subtle Energy Yoga (You're Doing It!)

Surprise! And congratulations! You may not know it yet, but you have already taken several major steps towards the understanding and practice of *Subtle Energy Yoga*!

By *subtle energy*, I mean internal energy flows that are subtle, but which are nevertheless present—and once you learn to detect them, they are far less subtle!

By *Subtle Energy Yoga*, I mean practices that generate those flows, and that stimulate your awareness of them—practices taken from Kundalini Yoga, Tantra Yoga, Raja Yoga, Ananda Yoga, Pranayama, Taiji (Tai Chi), and martial arts.

Many of those practices involve small muscular contractions that are all but invisible to the naked eye. To anyone watching, it may look as though you are just sitting—in your car, in the office, or meditating. But internally, a *lot* can be going on. That's what makes the practices *subtle*.

In this book, you have been introduced to several practices that do a great job of stimulating those flows:

1. **Sitting Asanas.**

   These forward bending exercises isolate each hip, giving it individual attention and quite possibly the best stretch it has ever had in its life! At least, that's if you grew up in the West, sitting in chairs.

   Perhaps the release of energy results from the location of the hips near the base of the spine. Or perhaps stretching the hips makes it easier to tilt your pelvis, which lets you straighten your back, stacking one vertebrae on top of another, producing the straight spine that allows energy to flow.

   Perhaps both factors play a role, or perhaps there is something else at play. For whatever reason, these practices are the most energy-releasing asanas I know! When I sit for meditation afterward, it feels like I am "coming home"—returning to the Bodhi tree to sit at the feet of my master and absorb all I can.

That's how powerful those sitting bends are—for me, at least. I hope you encounter similar feelings! Lacking flexibility, it took *years* before I encountered those energy flows using standard Yoga practices because, when sitting on the floor, my left hip was too tight to stretch the right hip, and vice versa.

Eventually, I got there—after a fashion. But it took a long time. And I still wasn't very flexible. So most of my progress was made at home, sitting on the edge of my futon!

But all that changed when I discovered the power of the *bench*. Once I did, things started happening, much more rapidly. My hope is that they will happen for you, too.

2. **Subtle Energy Enhancements**.
    You may have noticed that the basic and advanced *subtle energy enhancements* you learned for the sitting asanas include isometric exercises and other internal muscle contractions, such as the Healing "Tense-and-Relax" sequence that Yogananda taught to his students (and which I learned in Ananda's Raja Yoga series).

    Those enhancements can also be applied to other Yoga asanas, to a degree. But they find their greatest utility in the forward bends. And in the process, they stimulate energy flows so that a) They're stronger and, b) They're easier to recognize.

3. **"Sit Strengthener" Exercises**.
    These isotonic and isometric exercises contract the muscles at various points along the spine. In the process, they generate significant amounts of internal energy, and promote its flow.

If you are sitting happily between practice-segments, with a smile on your face, then I assure you that the energy is flowing!

If you are not already aware of those internal energy flows, I encourage you to open your awareness and look for them. Sit in meditation for a bit after doing those practices, and see what you feel. Be alert for waves of energy rising up, collecting at various energy points, and producing an internal expansion of those areas in the process.

You just may find that a door opens to a whole new world!

Learn More

If you are interested in learning more about energy-based Yoga and energy-flow meditation, read the remaining volumes in the *Subtle Energy Yoga*™ series. In those volumes, you'll learn:

- Even more about achieving the straight, upright spine that is a prelude to meditation.

- Subtle internal practices that stimulate those flows, including a set of subtle muscular contractions called *mudras* in Yoga, and another set called *bandhas*, which are actually two different words for different varieties of the same thing!

- Pranayama techniques and other techniques for stimulating those flows.

- A host of advanced practices, founded in the basics of mudras, bandhas, and pranayama, which take you to a whole new level.

- Meditation practices that use "mindfulness" as a starting point, and that end by lifting you into orbit!

Ask for them at your favorite bookstore and look for them on Amazon.

To learn more about the bench, visit yogaBench.TreeLight.com

For YouTube videos, see:

- The Yoga Bench Channel (use of the bench for sitting and for meditation)

- The Bench Yoga Channel (basic practices, possibly taught by a variety of teachers)

- The Subtle Energy Yoga Channel (deeper energy-flow practices)

To find out when Eric is giving a workshop on the subject, to hear about new books and articles as they are published, and for updates on the Yoga Meditation Bench, join the *Keys2Yoga* announcement group: groups.google.com/forum/#!forum/keys2yoga

Notes for Teachers

This chapter contains excerpts from a subsequent volume that discusses deeper aspects of teaching "internal energy flow" Yoga. These are the parts that pertain to a basic Bench Yoga class.

Setting Up Benches

When setting up benches for a Bench Yoga class, ensure that:

- Each bench has a base mat and a seat cushion.
  - Participants can move them out of the way for standard asanas, or use them.
  - But they should be there to allow for meditation *between* asanas.
- Each bench has 2 Yoga blocks, one on each side.
  - When doing seated bends, a participant can easily reach a block on either side. (For some bends, one side will be easier to access than the other.)
  - With two blocks, participants have one for each hand, which makes it easier for them to work their way down, or work their way back up.
- Ideally, each bench has a short support cushion under it.
  - For use in Leaning Vajrasana and Supported Warrior in Recline, among other things.
- There is enough space between benches for one block oriented sideways, and one oriented lengthways.
  - Sitting with both legs crossed on the bench, a large user needs an additional 7 inches of space on each side, for their knees.
  - Ideally, then, there is a total of 14 inches between benches.
  - Yoga blocks are 9 inches tall, 6 inches wide, and 4 inches deep. Use the 9-inch dimension and the 6-inch dimension to create a 15-inch gap, one more than is needed even for large users.

○   The distance between benches, front to back, depends on the type of class.

- For a Yoga asana class, there should be enough room in front of each bench to unroll a Yoga mat.

- For a meditation class, a half to a third of that space is sufficient.

○   For a mixed class:

- Set up in the middle with closely spaced benches, for "sitters". (Mats between those benches will be folded.)

- On the outside, set up with enough space for unfolded mats, for experienced Yoga practitioners who want to follow along on the mat when they can.

- An arrangement that looks like the one below can provide 10 benches with 6 folded mats and 4 unfolded:

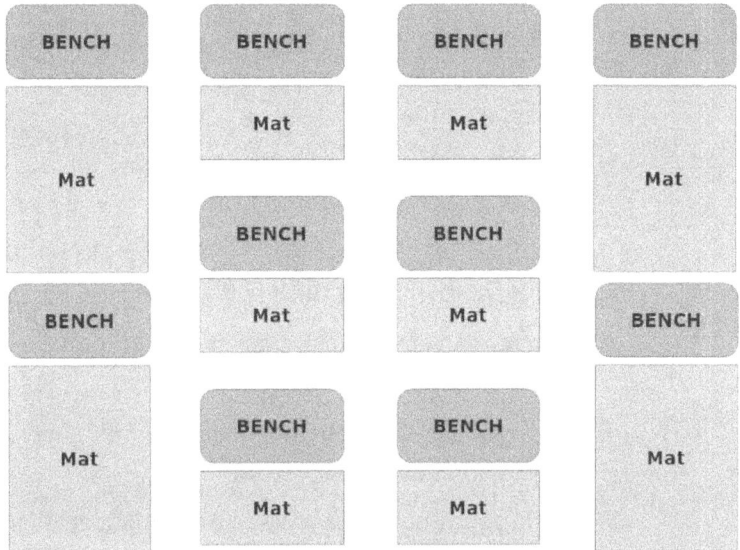

BENCH	BENCH	BENCH	BENCH
	Mat	Mat	
Mat			Mat
	BENCH	BENCH	
BENCH	Mat	Mat	BENCH
Mat	BENCH	BENCH	Mat
	Mat	Mat	

General Class Notes

Things to remind people of in most every class, unless you recognize the faces:

Late Arrivals

- If you come in late and the class is in the middle of a meditation practice, please do a standing meditation at the back, or sit down quietly and join in. Please wait for the meditation to finish before you set up mats, walk around, or make any noise!

  For more, see the sidebar on page 228:
  Late Arrivals Should be Quiet!

Listen to Your Inner Guidance

- Come out of a pose when you're ready.
- If you feel called to something different, by all means do that.
- Don't push yourself.
- Rejoin the flow the instructor is leading whenever you're ready.

Using the Bench

- If you are an experienced Yoga practitioner, or you can sit comfortably in Lotus Pose for 20 minutes or so, you may not need the bench. If you like, you can do the seated postures on the floor, preferably with a cushion under you. (But the advantage of using the bench is that when you tire, you can easily change positions!)
- In any case, you will probably find that the bench is the fastest route you can take to *achieve* the full Lotus position.

Late Arrivals Should be Quiet!

When meditating on your own, you'll find that you get to the point where external noises are only a minor distraction. In fact, you will eventually find that you can meditate easily in a crowded cafeteria or busy train station!

But when you are following a teacher in a *guided* meditation, it is critical to be focused solely on the instructions. For several reasons:

- In that setting, you are essentially in a self-induced meditative trance, where you are processing verbal instructions and converting them to images or sensations. External noises pull you right out of the internal experience!

- When you are following instructions in a class setting, it is rather to be expected that you are not yet so advanced that external noises will have no effect.

- A *constant* clamor in a cafeteria or train station, in effect, creates a background drone that can be as soothing as a waterfall. So continual noise is much less disruptive than a single, unexpected one.

- In a purely meditative state, your mind is drifting. Studies show that, after a sudden noise, a meditator's heart rate and respiration return to normal almost immediately. But *meditation* and *guided visualization* are not the same.

- People who are not engaged in the practice cannot necessarily be expected to behave any differently. So if a car alarm goes off or some other noise occurs, it can be relatively easily discounted.

- But when someone comes in to *participate* in the class and then *chooses* to disrupt the practice of others, they are either being unintentionally oblivious or intentionally rude—and at an internally-perceived *energy level*, that attitude of simply not caring is far more disruptive than the noise.

The goal, of course, is to grow into such a magnanimous spirit that even the unenlightened intentions of others are no longer disruptive. It's a great goal! But it's kind of like weight lifting. You need to spend a lot of time lifting smaller weights before you are prepared to tackle the big ones!

Asana Notes

Reminders to give to a class when you're teaching, or to yourself when practicing.

As needed:

- Be aware of whatever is tight. Alternately squeeze and relax it. Squeezing the muscle momentarily increases the tension, but gives you a degree of control. Relaxing the muscle then releases the tension.

- The Pause is Important

  - Pause as long between asanas for as long as you held the position, or until your breath recovers.

  - *Be aware* of the energy flows in your body. (Eventually. But at the start just "see how you feel".)

Technique notes:

- Yoga Interlace technique

  - When interlacing your fingers, *overlap* your pinkies instead of crossing them.

  - This is a surprisingly useful variation on the standard way of interlacing your fingers. It comes in handy in several circumstances.

- Using the hands for support

  - There are different ways of setting your hands on a Yoga Block to get a smoothly-varying progression of support heights.

  - For example, you can put your fingertips on the block, put middle knuckles on it, or make a fist and put the largest two knuckles on it. To go lower than that, you curl your fingers into your palm and put the flats of your fingers on the block, gradually lowering your palm until it reaches the block. (The variations are covered in depth in Volume 2 of this series.)

Meditation Notes

Reminders. Use as needed:

- ○   Review of body positions (back, head and neck, legs & arms, arms & hands, tongue)
- ○   Importance of sitting upright
- ○   How to sit on the ground (if hips allow it)
- ○   How to sit in a chair

How to manage discomfort (breath shift, squeeze/relax, cushion behind back)

Meditate with Eyes Open

When you're giving instructions to your students, it is important to have your eyes open, observing them. This detail is especially true when guiding a meditation.

Be Present, Maintain Volume

Naturally, you will be telling your students to softly close their eyes at the start of the meditation practice, and it is a perfectly sensible thing to close your eyes yourself, to set an example. But after a few seconds you should open them again, and be aware of your students.

For one thing, some people may need to shift their position to get comfortable. Especially if they are new, you may want to pause your instructions to give them a chance to do so.

But the more important reason for keeping your eyes open is *volume control.*

There is the perfectly reasonable feeling that you don't want to speak too loudly, for fear of disrupting the meditations that are in progress. So it makes perfect sense to modulate your volume a bit. But there are two things to know:

1. The students in class have already acclimated themselves to your normal speaking level. As long as you maintain that volume, they will not be disturbed.

2. After a period of silence, you will want to speak a little more softly,, so you break the silence gently. At the same time, you want your eyes open, to keep from going *too* low.

You see, there is a natural tendency to go into the meditation yourself, to feel it happening, and then to describe what's going on to your students as a form of "guided meditation" that gives them suggestions for what to do next, or where to put their attention.

That's *fine*, of course. It's perfectly fine to close your eyes in order to better "go within" and feel the inner guidance yourself, before passing it on to others. But when you do, there is a natural tendency for your voice to drop. To counteract that tendency, *open your eyes when you open your mouth* to pass on the instructions!

> **When you open your mouth to pass on guidance,**
> **open your eyes as well!**

There are several reasons for that principle:

1. With eyes closed, there is a tendency for your voice to keep getting softer and quieter—progressively more so as you go deeper.

    *   The problem, of course, is that as your voice goes softer, it becomes harder for others to hear!

    *   Ambient sounds that may have been virtually unnoticeable before (like the sounds of traffic drifting through a window, or a fan) are now closer to the level of your voice. They begin acting like *white noise* that drowns out your words.

    *   Students who may have been comfortably following your instructions before may suddenly—in the middle of their meditation—find it difficult to do so. They may even wind up *straining* to hear the instructions.

    *   Opening your eyes to speak helps to counteract that tendency.

2. If people are startled, you will see it. That feedback will help you determine the appropriate volume.

3. If a student puts their hand to their ear to indicate that they can't hear you, you'll never see it if your eyes are closed!

    •   That's pretty huge. Because the student has no good options!

    •   One option is to get your attention by speaking up—and in the process disrupt everyone else's meditation. No one who cares about others will ever do that.

    •   Another option is to get up and move closer—an action that will probably disrupt their meditation, and will almost certainly disrupt the meditations of those they pass.

    •   Their final option is to remain quiet, remain in place, and simply miss whatever it is you are saying. If they have their own practice, that tends to work out okay (if not great). They'll simply do what they normally do. But if they're just starting out, they can miss a lot—and possibly become disenchanted in the process.

It is natural not to want to disturb your students when they are meditating. But let me assure you: With your eyes closed, deep in meditation, you are no longer an accurate judge of how much volume is excessive! Trust me when I say that your normal speaking voice is fine! You'll probably get a *little* quieter, and that's fine. But a *lot* quieter is not a good idea.

Of course, loud noises really *are* jarring. But your normal speaking volume isn't. If your eyes are open when you're talking, you'll be more likely to maintain your normal volume.

To take away the fear of disturbing others, I would note that the Super-Learning technique that was popular in the 80's found that retention levels for information was incredible when they played adagio music to put you in a relaxed, alpha state (so you were, in effect, meditating), and you received short bursts of information intermittently.

You'd be relaxing for 2 or 3 minutes, if I recall correctly, and then get a 20- or 30-second burst. Or maybe it was a 15-second meditation and a 5-second burst. (Details are hazy.) Scanning brainwaves, they noticed that the EEG shot up as information came in, but then quickly settled down again to their former meditative levels.

That's what happens when you speak in a normal voice as people are meditating. They are, of course, highly alert and aware of the slightest sound in the environment. Or they have gone deep within. Either way, your words bring them back up towards normal consciousness for a bit, after which they quickly resume their former state.

So the instructions, when they are heard, are *effective*—not disruptive. And if they're not heard, I can tell you from personal experience that students feel a bit frustrated when they don't knowing what they are supposed to be doing! As I have done on occasion, they may quit trying to hear and simply perform your *own* practice! (Which is fine, if they already have a practice. But if they are neophytes, they're out of luck.)

How to Meditate with Eyes Open

When you're meditating with eyes open, you are gazing as though at the top of a distant mountain. You are not focused on any *one* thing in your field of vision. Rather, you are simultaneously aware of *everything* within it.

In martial arts, we called it "total awareness". In some psychological circles, it's called "wide-field awareness". You could also think of it as gazing *from* the third eye (rather than *at* it).

It can also be called "moving meditation", because it's something you can do while walking, running, or even just standing in line.

Whatever you call it, it's a state of relaxed readiness where you are totally aware of your surroundings.

> *Note:*
> You can practice it at stoplights, too. It improves reaction time like nothing else, so you move out quickly when the light changes. (I've been going into a state of "relaxed readiness" at stoplights for years, with steadily improving

reaction time. I would let my eyes take in the entire scene, without focusing anything in particular. It made a big difference. But recently I realized that I could center my consciousness *at the spiritual eye*, while doing that—which means that now, I meditate at stop lights, too!)

Going In and Out

It's perfectly fine to close your eyes and go within to get back into a meditative state yourself, so you can hear the intuition about what to do or say next, but as a teacher your job is to stay right at the boundary between meditation and a normal, awake state—just as the meditator's job is to stay right at the boundary of alpha-relaxation and theta-sleep, pulsing back and forth between the two states.

As an intermediary, functioning on behalf of your students, you need to do the same thing—pulsing back and forth between an internal quiet where you can hear your intuition, and then coming back to a more normal waking state when you vocalize those instructions for others.

Eventually, as you become really adept at teaching, you may acquire the ability to be fully meditating with eyes open! (Wouldn't that be grand? If you reach that point, come and teach me!) But until then, opening your eyes to speak helps ensure that your students hear you, and that you are aware of it when they don't. So when you close your eyes to go within, be sure to open them when relaying the instructions!

That practice may even help you to *develop* the ability to go deep within with your eyes open. It is a faculty worth developing, too, as it will undoubtedly take your practice to "the next level", where you are fully connected to your inner guide as you go about your daily life!

> *Note:*
> It can also be helpful to meditate with eyes half open, in the style of Lahiri Mahasaya. That mudra keeps you at the boundary between "within" (internal) and "without" (external)—right where you need to be, as a teacher!

Use Your Hand to Indicate Breath

There are times when it is difficult to talk! For example, when leading a breath exercise, it is difficult to talk during a period when you're supposed to be holding your breath! But if you *don't* hold your breath, it's hard to know how long to keep people there before allowing them to exhale.

The solution to the dilemma is to use a hand to represent the breath, and let people follow you with their eyes open, until they have the idea. (They can then close their eyes and follow their own rhythm.)

So your hand going up could represent an inhalation. Keeping it in place would represent holding the breath. Lowering would represent exhaling. For something like the Figure 8 Breath described in Volume 3 of this series, you could raise your hand up to your nose for a big inhalation, and up to mid-torso for a relaxed inhalation.

Use a Demonstrator to Show a Pose

Similarly, it can be difficult to talk when you are in the midst of a difficult pose. At such times, it's a good idea to get a proficient student (ideally, a prospective student) up in front of the class, so you can talk while they demonstrate.

Besides making it possible for you to speak, that practice gives the student a chance to get used to being in front of a class. Of course, that will inflate their ego a bit (as it does for you and me), and that's something we all have to work on. But at the same time, it's natural to be a little frightened when everyone is looking at you.

Being in front of a class without having to talk is a great way to get used to the situation, so it's not so fearful. The next step is to "interview" them, so they're doing a little speaking, and maybe sharing a story. That's something my martial arts master used to do all the time, both to bring people out of their shells and to inspire others.

That process helps to develop new teachers!

Maintaining Motivation

Maintaining motivation to teach is an interesting problem, for me.

At first, it's exciting. You're sharing things you know, and helping people improve. Whee! But after a while, it begins to get repetitious.

And that's where the problem is, for me. When I begin to repeat myself, I begin to get bored. And when I get bored I look for other things to do.

That was more of a problem when I was younger of course! I got bored really quickly back then, and needed to keep things new and exciting. But you reach a point in life where it would be nice if you didn't have to work so hard all the time!

At that point, it's good to have a skill you repeat without really thinking about it. And that's pretty well where I am today.

Still, I'm alert to the problem of dwindling motivation, by dint of repetition. It's a problem worth being prepared for.

I see several possible solutions for that problem:

1. Teach a series of Workshops

2. Share Your Practice

3. Connect with Students

The remainder of this section discusses each of those solutions, in turn.

Teach a Series of Workshops

One possible solution for me (as author of this book), is to travel around the country giving a series of workshops based on the book. There would be enough repetition in the process to develop skill, but the sequence would have an ending.

Then it will be time the publish the next book in the series, like Wayne Dyer used to do, or even give the series again after a year or two have passed, depending on how much people are clamoring for it.

For someone who is launching their own career, a similar idea would be to give workshops around your city or state, based on this book, perhaps in combination with other sources of inspiration.

At the back of the workshop, you could have a table with books and Yoga equipment for sale, to help people to develop their own practice.

As always, the key to making something like that work is marketing! Somehow, the workshops need a recognizable "brand", and the word needs to get out.

One possible solution is for a series of teachers to give workshops under the same brand—say, "Subtle Energy Yoga", for instance, or "Bench Yoga". Each workshop would then be slightly different, by virtue of the person giving it, which would make it interesting and informative for people who have taken a workshop previously, as well as those coming to it for the first time.

Those teachers, in turn, could potentially go around the country teaching a series of workshops, and experiencing new territories in the process. It's something to consider, at least.

Share Your Practice

Another way to prevent boredom is simply to share your current practice! Since my practice keeps evolving, each class or workshop will tend to be slightly different from the one before.

If you follow that pattern, the class or workshop you teach this year will probably be a *lot* different from the one you taught last year.

Connect with Students

Another possible mechanism for maintaining a continuing motivation is to really *connect* with your students.

These days, my asana practice is one long meditation. It feels great. Every time I come up for a pose I experience a release of energy and have a joyful meditation—to the point that it has become somewhat addictive!

If I can create the kind of rapport with my students that allows me to feel that experience *vicariously,* then the teaching process could become as joyful—and as potentially addictive—as my personal practice.

Were that to happen, repetition while teaching wouldn't matter, any more than repetition matters in my personal practice—because each time, I would be experiencing the joyful energy that makes it worthwhile!

And to the degree I can connect well enough to really *know* my students, I can customize the class so it aligns more closely to their needs.

A New Paradigm

In the current teaching paradigm, everyone comes to class and does the same thing. Students are generally encouraged to adjust an asana to match their ability, but except for when someone goes into child pose to rest, it is pretty much the case that everyone is doing the same thing all that time.

In that model, the teacher is constantly giving instructions. There is little scope for a student to sit in meditation for a period of time between asanas, or to learn to let their inner voice direct their practice.

On the other hand, a group setting provides a lot of intention-energy that sanctifies the location, making it conducive to meditation and a personal practice. So, while you have more freedom to vary your practice at home, there are definite benefits to a class setting—not the least of which is the opportunity to take time away from your normal distractions and dwell in an environment that is conducive to personal growth.

What if it were possible to get the best of both worlds?

In a boxing gym or mixed-martial arts (MMA) gym, everyone works on their own. They get advice from roving instructors but, as when they are lifting weights, it is up to the student to do the work.

A meditative Yoga-center can be run on that model. During set times, the center would be open for use, with benches and Yoga mats in place. During that time, people could come and pursue their personal practice in a nurturing environment.

For guidance, a series of poses could be posted each day—one for beginners, one for intermediates, and one for advanced. A student could take a copy of the one they want to follow—or a couple of different ones, to mix and match.

A roving instructor could then offer guidance when it seems appropriate—talking quietly, but not exactly whispering. (Because any speech that is positive and purposeful—as well as respectful—is unlikely to bother those who are meditating.)

Normal classes can be given as well, of course. But the focus in those classes can be less about leading a practice, and more about picking a few poses and going into the finer points for advanced practitioners, with easier variations for people who are building up to that point.

Attending such a class would be much like going on a meditation retreat—but at a time and for a duration that fits conveniently into the student's lifestyle.

Becoming Certified

At some point, an organization will be needed to manage a certification process. But there isn't one, as yet. (Good news! Ground floor opportunity! Easiest time to get on board!)

Even when an organization exists, the certification process should be simple, I think:

1. You attend enough classes to have been exposed to the complete set of concepts.

2. A qualified representative of the organization attends a class of yours.

    a. It is *not* required that you teach everything, exactly as it was taught you, and *only* those things.

    b. Hopefully, instead, you are bringing your own flavor and what you have learned from others into the mix.

    c. What *is* required is that you reflect the spirit and fundamental ideas of the meditative Subtle Energy Yoga technique.

3. After attending your class and feeling uplifted and connected, the representative reports back, and you are issued a certificate!

Of course, at the moment, there is no organization. And there is only one representative: Yours truly! But stress not. If you're already teaching Yoga, you are undoubtedly a more *experienced* teacher. You're probably even a *better* teacher. So if you learned the powerful ideas and techniques presented in this book, you could be receiving a Certificate of Certification forthwith!

The Rationale for Certification

Some sort of minimal certification is obviously required to teach this style of Yoga, just so prospective students know what you're doing—and so the concept of "Subtle Energy Yoga" (or "Bench Yoga") remains identifiable, rather than being applied to a multiple of different practices.

Those requirements are minimal, though, because the whole idea is to be flexible, rather than rigid—and there are undoubtedly many who have already advanced along this path! Mostly, then, they need a recognizable brand-name to teach under, so people know they will be improving their meditation practice, and their lives.

And that is the reason for preserving the brand! The Western world needs a more meditative style of Yoga. And it needs to be easy to find! The brand makes it identifiable. And, as it grows more popular, it becomes a style of Yoga that more people *want* to teach.

Resources

Yoga Bench and Accessories

When you purchase a bench at yogaBench.TreeLight.com, accessories increase your discount. So that is the most cost-effective way to get the accessories you need. But you can also order accessories from Amazon, or direct from the manufacturers:

- **Base Pad:**
  Amazon: Bean Products Zabuton, 24 x 24 x 2"
  Direct: BeanProducts.com

- **Seat Cushion:**
  Amazon: Bean Products Rectangular Bolster, 24" x 12" x 6"
  Direct: BeanProducts.com

- **Support Cushion:**
  Amazon: Gayo Meditation Cushion, 10 x 15 x 5" (if available)
  Amazon: YogaAccessories Cotton Meditation Pillow, 15 x 11 x 5"
  Direct: YogaAccessories.com

YouTube Instructionals

How to Stop a Calf Cramp in Seconds (YouTube), by Dr. Marco Caravaggio
https://www.youtube.com/watch?v=Xenoxxxn3rM
Immediate relief from a cramp!

Preparation for Lotus, by David Keil
A great preparatory sequence for Lotus Pose. Beginners will find it easier to do it on the bench. Advanced intermediates will find it fine on the ground, as in the video. Either way, this is one inspired video that shows you how the limbs need to be rotated to make the pose achievable.

Working with the Knee in Lotus, by David Keil
This video is a bit more detailed. It makes the great point that where most people experience pain is in the inside corner of the knee. That was a major inspiration for the Limb Rotation Sequence that helps you grow into advanced poses.

Primal Posture by Esther Gokhale
This short talk describes "primal posture", with great pictures depicting people exhibiting it—effortlessly, and without fanfare. (Spoiler: The *key* to being upright and *relaxed* is to put your behind *behind* you. The resulting pelvic tilt puts your mid- and upper-back upright, while remaining relaxed.)

Teaching Traditions

Bihar School of Yoga
The school founded by Swami Shivananda Saraswati. Teaches *Shivananda Yoga*—a "wisdom tradition" Yoga that relies heavily on ancient texts collected and written up by Patanjali. One of its graduates is Swami Asanganand Saraswati, mentioned below. Another is Sunyata Saraswati, who along with co-founder Bodhi Avinasha, created Ipsalu Tantra Yoga, described next.

Ipsalu Tantra Yoga
An "energy flow" tradition that focuses on chakras and energy work— in other words, *Kriya Yoga*. Although sexuality is not its main focus, it does not shy away from it, either. So it encourages intimacy and embraces sexuality as part of the practitioner's growth towards enlightenment and bliss.

Jung SuWon
The school of martial arts founded by Grandmaster Tae Yun Kim. Essentially, an "internal" form of Tae Kwan Do, where the goal is internal growth, rather than competitive prowess. Focuses on heart-centered meditation and growth through internal discipline. Her philosophy is best captured in her book, Seven Steps to Inner Power.

The Art and Science of Raja Yoga (book), by Swami Kriyananda
A guide to awakening the energy centers at the top of the spine, inviting energy to rise. It's a perfect companion to Kundalini Yoga, which generates energy at the bottom of the spine and moves it upwards. In between, of course, a great deal of "emotional clearing" is generally needed to clear the emotional blockages that interfere with energy movement. But when everything works in harmony, the results are uplifting, illuminating, and elevating!

Ananda
Their Northern California location in Palo Alto is where I undertook the Raja Yoga course I found so illuminating. One of the schools that keeps Yogananda's teachings alive, along with the Self Realization Fellowship in Southern California.

Swami Asanganand Saraswati
A Yoga *Shibir* is a free workshop (donations-encouraged) with introductions to the finer points of Shivananda Yoga, and living the Yoga lifestyle.

Chair Yoga

Additional ideas and inspirations for your Bench Yoga practice.

Discovering Chair Yoga (DVD), with Steve Wolf
Great if you enjoy following a DVD to practice.

Chair Vinyasa: Yoga Flow for Every Body (book), by Delia Quigley
Nicely written and illustrated. I have sticky-tab bookmarks all over it.

A Chair for Yoga (book), by Eyal Shifroni
A complete guide to Iyengar Yoga practice with a chair. Comprehensive and authoritative.

Chair Yoga (book), by Kristin McGee
Good poses and sequences.

All I Need is This Chair Yoga (book), by Wilma Carter
A basic, fun introduction.

Tai Chi!

The benefits of muscle-squeezing exercises have already been mentioned. Tai Chi (or *Taiji*, in its original spelling) is a gentle, effective form of exercise that complements Yoga nicely.

You can do it sitting on a bench as an extra-gentle way to encourage energy flows, or do a standing version to get more work for the legs. Here are a couple of resources to aid in that practice.

Tai Chi in a Chair, by Cynthia Quarta
> Another form of exercise you can do on the bench—with your back in the perfect position!

Step by Step Tai Chi for Seniors, by Dejun Jue
> To round out your Yoga and sitting Tai Chi program, it is helpful to do things that strengthen the legs (improving your balance in the process). I've studied Taiji (the original Chen form, with has martial-arts applications), and I like it. But I'm daunted by the long, repetitive forms which—despite their repetitions—still tend to work only one side of the body! This book contains a sequence that is long enough to cover a lot of ground, but without a lot of duplication. It is also short enough to be mastered quickly, and short enough to learn and perform on each side!

Yoga, Health, and Healing

How to Meditate: A Step-by-Step Guide (book), by Jyotish Novak.
> Terrific introduction to meditation, with a wealth of tips, practices, and reports on scientific research.

Science of Breath (book), by Swami Rama
> Although the importance of breath and deep-breathing practices is now taken for granted, in its day it was understood by only a few. (The same situation exists for the effect of electricity and magnetism, today! This book explains the science and the effects of deep breathing practices.

Science of Breath (book), by Swami Ramacharaka
A short, republished classic from 1904 that details Yogic breathing practices

The Yoga System of Health and Relief from Tension (book), by Yogi Vithaldis
Small, fantastic book that introduces Yoga asanas (postures), plus pranayama, meditation, and internal cleansing practices.

The Ultimate Beginner's Guide to Yoga
https://hobbyhelp.com/yoga/
A comprehensive online guide to choosing the right style of Yoga for you and the equipment you need, plus a variety of poses to get you started.

Easy Yoga for Seniors (VHS Tape), by Pat Laster (available now on YouTube)
Although old, this is one great video. The pacing is superb, with many moments for meditation, and it has a good introduction to the 3-Part Yogic Breath (aka "Complete Breath"). It's a great video everyone can use together—an experienced practitioner can always do more difficult variations on the postures, much more easily than, say, a beginner can figure out how to make hard poses easier! (Since the 1994 copyright lapsed in 2011, and since the "Video Vacation" company no longer exists as far as I can tell, I uploaded it to YouTube.)

The Ultimate Guide to the Face Yoga Method (book), by Fumiko Takatsu
A practice that removes wrinkles and keeps you looking young!

Science

Health Benefits of Rocking Chairs (article)

https://www.utilitydesign.co.uk/blog/health-benefits-of-rocking-chairs/

Rocking is good for you!

Progressive muscle relaxation

https://www.sciencedirect.com/topics/medicine-and-dentistry/progressive-muscle-relaxation

The history and science of consciously tensing (squeezing) a muscle in order to relax it.)

Lymphatic System: Facts, Functions, and Diseases

https://www.livescience.com/26983-lymphatic-system.html

A good article with a video and a large, descriptive "info graphic" that summarizes what there is to know in a nutshell.

Lymphatic System

https://en.wikipedia.org/wiki/Lymphatic_system

A nice introduction to the operation and effects of the Lymph System.

Super-Learning, by Sheila Ostrander

Quiet, meditative music coupled with short-bursts of information at intervals produces near-total memory recall! The intervals need to be long enough that you get back to a drifting, meditative state. The information bursts need to be short enough that they don't pull you completely out of it. Get the timing right, and learning becomes a powerfully calming practice that is at the same time extremely effective.

YouTube   U

My collection of science videos covering the Electric Universe model, plasma physics, the nature of magnetic fields, and more.

BioElectricity

BioEnergetics (PDF)
Deep physiology: How cells generate and utilize energy.
http://www.nmr.sinica.edu.tw/~thh/lectures/Biophysics/Chap_3Bio
energetics.pdf

The Body Electric (book), by Dr. Robert Becker
Comprehensive review of the entire history of research into biological
electricity, plus explanations of his research and a survey of current
trends. A fascinating read that shows how success treating some all-
too-common diseases caused the chemical model of the body to be
adopted, in lieu of the electrical model. But both models clearly have
their place—and the electrical model has a much better track record
when it comes to "lifestyle problems" like cancer and heart disease.

PEMF: The 5th Element of Health (book), by Bryant Meyers
Readable and inspirational, this book studies the use of magnetic fields
for healing, based on the principle of resonance with the fields
produced by a Pulsed ElectroMagnetic Frequency (PEMF) device that
operates at the frequencies produced by the earth. (One of the reasons
why, along with air and sunshine, we feel so much better when
outdoors.)

PH and Voltage (YouTube), by Dr. Jerry Tennant
This 24-minute introduction is the place to start, to investigate Dr.
Tennant's concepts. Ties together body electricity, Chi meridians, and
chakras. (Dr. Tennant's device works by directly stimulating the body
with electrically-generated energy.)

Jerry Tennant: Healing is Voltage: The Physics of Emotions (YouTube)
A 48-minute video that goes deeper into the subject. Likens muscles
to a stack of batteries.

Healing is Voltage: On/Off switches for Cancer (YouTube), Jerry
Tenant, M.D.
Shows how cell membranes act as batteries. See the picture at 30:53
for a nice list of lifestyle elements that drain energy or add energy—

quite literally, by way of taking or giving electrons.

At 10:58, he describes the *piezoelectric effect* of muscles, where the effect of stretching and squeezing (stress on the material) products electricity. As explained at 17:40, the generated electrons are then pushed through the *fascia* that surrounds muscle tissue—a *semiconductor* that is a one-way conductor of electricity. If his ideas are true, it explains the increased internal energy flows experienced in muscle-squeezing practices, and how the energy supplied by sunlight at the level of skin can be moved into internal tissues.

Healing is Voltage (book), by Dr. Jerry Tennant

Dr. Tennant's book on the subject. He does a great job of explaining everything related to his theories, but when it comes to his theories themselves, he simply makes statements, without citing evidence or research. That makes the book somewhat less than fully convincing. (In many ways, his introductory video is better.) Nevertheless, my sense is that he is on to something.

https://www.amazon.com/Healing-Voltage-Handbook-Jerry-Tennant/dp/1453649166/

YouTube U

A collection of videos covering the Electrical Universe (EU), plasma theory and experiments, plus the true properties of magnetism. Eye-opening   explanations,   backed   by   experimental   evidence!

About the Author

Eric Armstrong has spent 30 years in spiritual pursuits, including Hatha Yoga, training and teaching martial arts, exploring Tantra, and studying Raja Yoga. A former athlete and coach, he brings Western sensibilities to Eastern spirituality, creating a system that is at once deep and practical—one that focuses on the essence of Yoga: *Samadhi*, or a blissful sense of enlightenment.

A former volleyball player and coach (and runner, and soccer player), Eric indulges his competitive instincts with a game of pool, and the occasional round of golf. (He *wants* to treat them as a meditation—but finds it difficult to maintain equanimity in the face of the inevitable frustrations!)

He lives in California, in San Francisco's South Bay.

Contact Eric through his website: http://treelight.com

Follow him on Twitter: @ericTreeLight

Support him on Patreon: http://patreon.com/ericArmstrong

TreeLight PenWorks

TreeLight.com was founded by Eric Armstrong in 1997 as a free-information site devoted to all aspects of health: fitness, nutrition, spiritual, social, and societal. Independently owned and operated, it exists to provide useful information to the public at large. (It also provides links to recommended products at Amazon.com, which produce a modicum of income, as is the case with the eBook edition of this book.)

TreeLight PenWorks ("Unique Perspectives, Clearly Explained") is an extension of the website that was formed to provide books like this one, to provide deeper, in-depth treatment of selected topics in the areas of Golf, Yoga, Health, Fitness, and Political Reform.

For more titles available from TreeLight PenWorks, visit TreeLight.com/books.

www.ingramcontent.com/pod-product-compliance
Lightning Source LLC
LaVergne TN
LVHW051500080426
835509LV00017B/1835